NEURO-OTOLOGICAL EXAMINATION

with Special Reference to Equilibrium Function Tests

TAKUYA UEMURA, M.D.

Professor of Otolaryngology
Tokyo Women's Medical College, Tokyo, Japan

JUN-ICHI SUZUKI, M.D.

Professor of Otolaryngology
Teikyo University School of Medicine, Tokyo, Japan

JIRO HOZAWA, M.D.

Associate Professor of Otolaryngology
Tohoku University School of Medicine, Sendai, Japan

STEPHEN M. HIGHSTEIN, M.D.

Associate Professor of Neuroscience
Albert Einstein College of Medicine, Bronx, New York, U.S.A.

UNIVERSITY PARK PRESS
BALTIMORE AND LONDON

IGAKU SHOIN LTD. TOKYO

Library of Congress Cataloging in Publication Data
Main entry under title:

Neuro-otological examination.

    1. Vestibular function tests. 2. Neurologic examination.
I. Uemura, Takuya, 1971–
RF123.N48   617.8'8   76–6498
ISBN 0-8391-0887-7

PUBLISHERS
© First Edition, 1977 by IGAKU SHOIN LTD., 5-24-3 Hongo, Bunkyo-ku, Tokyo.
    Rights in the United States of America, the Dominion of Canada, Latin America and Europe
    including the United Kingdom granted to
    UNIVERSITY PARK PRESS: Chamber of Commerce Building, Baltimore, Maryland 21202.

Printed in Japan. Composed and printed by Gakujutsu Tosho Printing Co., Ltd., Tokyo and
bound by Kojima Binding Co., Ltd., Tokyo. The photographic engravings for the illustrations
were made by Gakujutsu Photoengraving Co., Ltd., Tokyo.

Foreword

Twenty years ago vestibular function tests were the only standard examination for patients complaining of vertigo. Recently, however, it has been generally agreed that vestibular tests should be only a portion of the examination related to equilibrium function. Since vertigo or dizziness is one of the subjective symptoms of vestibular dysfunction it seems most important to obtain some objective correlates of this complaint. Many different methods of analysis have therefore been adopted for qualitatively and quantitatively evaluating equilibrium dysfunction. Not only the location of the underlying pathology but also the nature of the lesion must be determined in order to effect a correct diagnosis and treatment. It is thus apparent that traditional vestibular tests do not suffice: improvement in the currently available examinations and development of new techniques are strongly needed. Further, the results of such functional analyses including audiologic tests must be interpreted on the basis of a systemic neurological understanding. The term "neuro-otology" is based on this concept.

The authors of this book are all actively engaged in research in this newly expanding field of neuro-otology and their original contributions in this area have been quite eminent. The current status of our understanding of neuro-otology is delineated in this volume and a prospectus for future research is also noted.

It is my pleasure to recommend this epoch-making volume to specialists all over the world. I am convinced that this publication will contribute significantly to the development of neuro-otology.

MASANORI MORIMOTO, M.D.
Professor and Director
Department of Otolaryngology
Faculty of Medicine, Kyoto University
Kyoto, Japan

Foreword

The vestibular system includes a complex of central connections which form various pathways and reflexes influencing three major systems; the oculomotor, the somatic motor, and the autonomic nervous systems. The cerebellum and the cerebrum have also been shown to be connected with the vestibular system. The conventional vestibular function tests previously employed, however, have been centered around investigating the peripheral vestibular organs, while the relationship of these organs to the brain as an entity has been rather neglected.

During the past twenty years, the fundamental significance of vestibular function tests has been re-evaluated and this has given rise to several new methods of testing. The development of these modern methods has been supported by the progress in our understanding of the anatomy, physiology and pharmacology of the brain. Internists, neurologists and neurosurgeons have also contributed to this development. Modern equilibrium function tests endeavor to assess the equilibrium state of the whole human body without reference to a particular set of organs and should not be bound by the framework of a particular medical subspeciality. The scope of equilibrium function tests has thus been greatly enlarged and this is why the title of this monograph "neuro-otology" was chosen in preference to the title "vestibular function tests".

This book aims at clarifying the significance of each equilibrium function test. The clinical interpretation of the test results is provided and the step-by-step explanation of procedures for important test methods are explained. The rich supply of clinical material covered in the book will also assist in gaining an understanding of the clinical application of the tests.

I fully expect to see this book take its place as a classic in the field of neuro-otology.

ICHIRO KIRIKAE, M.D.
Professor Emeritus
Faculty of Medicine, University of Tokyo;
Professor and Director,
Department of Otolaryngology
Jichi Medical School
Tochigi, Japan

Preface

In 1968 the "Neurotological Examination with Special Reference to Vestibular Function Tests" was published by Drs. T. Uemura, J. Suzuki and J. Hozawa in Japan. It was based on the contents of the symposium on the "Problems in utilizing equilibrium function tests as routine tests" held at the 67th Annual Scientific Meeting of the Japan Oto-Rhino-Laryngological Society on May 5, 1966. The book received a wide welcome not only by otologists but also by neurologists, neurosurgeons and others. This encouraged us to promote publication of the English edition.

A considerable portion of the book has been rewritten and the chapter on the neuro-logic examination by Dr. S. M. Highstein has been added as this examination is indispensable for obtaining the correct diagnosis in patients with vertigo and/or disequilibrium. The standardization of the neuro-otological examination has, however, not been completed. Parts of the examination are still being performed by individual physicians according to their personal experience and preference, and are not necessarily based on current knowledge of vestibular mechanisms. It is our hope that this book will stimulate discussion on many of these individual viewpoints and will contribute to the synthesis of a standard method for the neuro-otological examination.

We wish to express our sincere thanks to many friends and colleagues, without whose cooperation this book could not have been completed. We are particularly grateful to Drs. M. Morimoto and I. Kirikae for their contribution of forewords, and also to Dr. B. Cohen, Professor of Neurology at the Mount Sinai School of Medicine of The City University of New York, for his valuable suggestions and advice. The authors would like to express their gratitude to Ms. R. Sekhar for editorial assistance. Gratitude is also due to the cooperation and assistance of the staff of the Igaku Shoin Ltd.

T. U.

Contents

I

Introduction

Selection of the Test Methods in the Neuro-Otological Examination

The neuro-otological examination is performed for the purpose of diagnosis and to evaluate the course of treatment. As it is usually necessary to compare the results of repeated examinations, a small number of carefully selected tests should be employed in order to efficiently and accurately obtain the optimum amount of information.

Before any special tests are employed a routine medical history and physical examination should be performed. The examiner then evaluates the patient's symptoms with reference to the vestibular system if indicated and tries to reach a tentative diagnosis. Further appropriate diagnostic tests are then employed to determine the location, extent, and etiology of the pathologic process.

The following three conditions concerning the location of the process should be satisfied.

1) differentiation between vestibular and non-vestibular disorders
2) differentiation between peripheral and central vestibular disorders
3) differentiation between the affected and normal sides.

1), 2) and 3) can usually be accomplished by performing a series of clinical examinations including a basic neurologic examination. Next, an attempt should be made to evaluate the extent and etiology of the lesion. Laboratory tests are often helpful in this regard. An example of the procedure is listed in Table 1.

Indications for the Neuro-Otological Examination

All diseases connected with vertigo and dizziness*, equilibrium disturbance, tinnitus and deafness may be referred to the otologist and *should be studied by the neuro-otological examination.*

VERTIGO AND DIZZINESS OF VESTIBULAR AND NON-VESTIBULAR ORIGIN

When the origin of an equilibrium disturbance is in the vestibular system, it is called a vestibular equilibrium disturbance, and is differentiated from a non-vestibular disturbance. Dizziness of ocular origin or psychogenic dizziness, usually continuous rather than episodic, belongs to the latter category of illness. The neuro-otological examination is useful in differentiating a vestibular disturbance from a non-vestibular disturbance i.e. positive results indicating vestibular dysfunction may be taken as synonymous with vestibular dis-

---

* The words vertigo and dizziness are often used interchangeably; however vertigo implies a sensation of turning which is not necessarily present in dizziness. Neither word has any etiologic implications.

Table 1   An approach to the patient.   When a patient comes to the doctor with complaints of vertigo, tinnitus and hearing loss, the following procedures are performed in order to determine the cause and extent of the illness, and to follow the effects of any treatment which is necessary.

Patient
1. *History-taking*
2. *General physical examination*
3. *Diagnostic tests*

a. Ascertain the location of the illness (Differential diagnosis, peripheral or central?).

Appropriate tests:
Hearing test,
Spontaneous-, positional-, and positioning nystagmus test,
Self-recording cupulometry,
Caloric test,
Optokinetic nystagmus test
Neurologic examination

b. Ascertain the cause and extent of the illness

Appropriate tests:
Test for focal infection (oral cavity, teeth, paranasal sinuses and tonsils).
Otoscopy and X-ray examination of temporal bone.
Laboratory examination (Autonomic nervous function).
More detailed investigation of results of equilibrium and neurologic examinations.
Angiography or encephalography in cases with suspected endocranial lesion.

Diagnosis and determination of *course* of treatment. For example, the diagnosis of Ménière's disease is established.

4. *Serial tests* conducted after the beginning of treatment(Evaluation of effects of treatment and estimation of prognosis).

Appropriate tests:
Spontaneous-, positional- and positioning tests,
Rotation test,
Optokinetic nystagmus test and eye-tracking test, hearing test.

turbance.   If the results of all neuro-otological examinations are equivocal, a psychogenic or other disease process may be suspected.

PERIPHERAL AND CENTRAL VESTIBULAR DISTURBANCES

When the origin of an equilibrium disorder is in the labyrinth or the vestibular nerve, the disorder is called a peripheral vestibular disturbance and may be differentiated from a central disturbance, which originates from malfunction of the vestibular nuclei or the higher central neural pathways.

PERIPHERAL VESTIBULAR DISTURBANCE

1. Diseases Accompanied by Cochlear Symptoms
a. Ménière's disease
In order to diagnose Ménière's disease, the following conditions must be satisfied. Vertiginous attacks accompanied by nausea or vomiting occur repeatedly and the recurrence of the attack is associated with the exacerbation of cochlear symptoms.   In most cases, unilateral sensory-neural hearing loss is documented by audiometry, and the alternate binaural loudness balance test (ABLB) or Békésy's audiometry shows the recruitment phenomenon.   Peripheral vestibular disturbance is confirmed by equilibrium function tests.   All cranial nerves except for the VIIIth nerve are unimpaired.   X-ray of the temporal bone and otoscopic findings are normal.   The Wassermann test reaction is negative (refer to Case Studies–1, p. 138).

b. Acute labyrinthosis (or vestibulopathy) with sudden deafness

The vertiginous attack is accompanied by unilateral severe deafness. The process of exacerbation is so rapid that it is also called an apoplectic form of Ménière's disease. This attack, however, may have a different pathogenesis from Ménière's disease and is thought to be caused by a virus infection or insufficient blood circulation in the inner ear (refer to Case Studies–4, p. 144).

c. Drug intoxication

Hair cells of the inner ear are sensitive to the toxicity of drugs such as salicylates, quinine, streptomycin, kanamycin, and some other antibiotics. Labyrinthine function is influenced by intoxication, and cochlear and vestibular symptoms may be produced.

d. Virus infection

Herpes zoster oticus (Hunt's syndrome), presumably caused by viral inflammation of the geniculate ganglion, is accompanied by facial paralysis and auditory and vestibular symptoms. Mumps deafness is rarely associated with vertigo.

e. Specific inflammation

Syphilitic labyrinthitis has Ménière-like symptoms. A positive Wassermann's test may differentiate between the two diseases. Cogan's syndrome, sarcoidosis and other so-called collagen diseases may exhibit evidence of vestibulo-cochlear involvement.

f. Acoustic trauma

The relation between intense noise and vertigo is known as Tullio's phenomenon. Sensory deafness caused by acoustic trauma is often accompanied by dizziness or unsteadiness. The audiogram may show a characteristic high tone notch (C_5 dip).

2. Vertigo Accompanied by Otitis Media (Vertigo Secondary to Ear Surgery)

Vertigo and disturbed equilibrium are often found in cases of otitis media, specifically in cholesteatoma otitis. In these cases, the following causes should be considered: perilabyrinthitis, labyrinthine fistula, serous or purulent labyrinthitis, and endocranial complications (cerebellar abscess) (refer to Case Studies–2, p. 140).

A peripheral vestibular disturbance is also common after ear surgery. The semicircular canal fenestration operation or stapedectomy for otosclerosis especially may be accompanied by long lasting vertigo.

3. Vertigo Induced by a Cervical Cause

When transient episodes of vertigo are induced by turning the head and neck, a cervicovestibular syndrome (Hozawa, 1973) may be suspected. When the head is rotated and the neck extended, the vertebral artery can be compressed by a spondylotic spur. This mechanical pressure on the vertebral artery stimulates the perivascular sympathetic nerve plexus and induces vasoconstriction of the blood vessels of the inner ear, resulting in a peripheral vestibular disturbance. In such cases, spondylosis deformans or kinking of the vertebral artery can often be demonstrated by X-ray studies. The cochlea is not usually affected in this syndrome (refer to Case Studies–5, p. 146).

If vertebral arterial flow is compromised by chronic cervical osteoarthritis, transient vertigo accompanied by focal transient neurologic deficits due to medullary ischemia may be experienced.

4. Vertigo without Cochlear Symptoms

Vestibular neuronitis (Dix-Hallpike, 1952) and positional vertigo of the benign paroxysmal type belong to this category (refer to Case Studies–3, p. 142). The etiology of the first is obscure but the latter is thought to be caused by an otolithic lesion and is characterized by transient nystagmus and vertigo which is induced by a specific head position.   Acute viral labyrinthitis and epidemic vertigo, which is sometimes accompanied by brainstem encephalitis, are usually included in this category.

5.   Vertigo of Unknown Etiology

There are a considerable number of cases, in which the causes of vertigo cannot be elucidated, although the results of equilibrium function tests and the absence of evidence of neighboring brainstem deficits are strongly suggestive of a peripheral vestibular disturbance. These include patients complaining of repeated attack of vertigo without accompanying auditory symptoms or a single attack of vertigo accompanied by auditory symptoms. We suggest that a tentative diagnosis of "aural vertigo of unknown etiology" be assigned to these patients.

CENTRAL VESTIBULAR DISTURBANCE

1.   Cerebellopontine Lesion
a.   Acoustic tumor

When unilaterally progressive deafness is accompanied by symptoms such as equilibrium disturbance, unilateral headache, and facial paresthesia, an acoustic tumor should be suspected.   The main findings of the neuro-otological examination are as follows:
1)   Retrocochlear deafness is verified by hearing tests: 2)   hypoexcitability or loss of excitability in the affected labyrinth is observed by the caloric test and 3) gaze and positional nystagmus are characteristic.   Bruns' nystagmus is often observed in the "brain tumor" stage.   Positional nystagmus is mainly of the direction-changing type (NYLÉN's type I) and vertical or diagonal nystagmus can be elicited during the positioning test.   If the disease has progressed, examination of the gait may reveal staggering, reeling or lurching. As a rule, the gait deviates towards the affected side.   The spontaneous arm-tonus reaction may also be found as the arm on the affected side sinks down when the patient is asked to close his eyes and hold his arms out in front of him.   A characteristic change in the optokinetic nystagmus pattern test can also be observed, but the so-called "reversion phenomenon" is not revealed by self-recording cupulometry.   This phenomenon is observed exclusively when a labyrinthine lesion is present (refer to "The rotation test", p. 80).

Cerebellar and cranial nerve (V, VI, VII, IX) symptoms and signs are observed in the "brain tumor" stage.   Morphological changes of the internal auditory canal or the pyramis are often demonstrated by X-ray (refer to X-ray Studies, Fig. 95, p. 121).

b.   Other diseases

All tumors or pachymeningitis in the cerebellopontine angle display symptoms similar to acoustic tumors.

2.   Lesion in the Brainstem ro the Cerebellum
a.   Vertebral-basilar insufficiency

Symptoms and signs resulting from interference with the blood flow in the vertebral-basilar artery and its branches vary according to the site of the stenosis or occlusion, but do not always correspond exactly to any anatomical defect which may be demonstrable by neuroradiology or neuropathology.   Rather, dysfunction results from the physiological defect in blood flow which is dependent upon the collateral circulation, blood pressure, heart rate and many other variables.   For example, occlusion of one vertebral artery may or may not result in any noticeable central nervous system dysfunction.

The most common manifestations of vertebral-basilar insufficiency are transient dizzy spells, drop attacks, paresthesias of the face (especially perioral), or of one side of the face and body, decrease in vision, double vision, slurred speech, and ataxia. If a history of recurrent episodes of vertigo is accompanied by such transient neurologic complaints, the physician should be alerted that dysfunction of the central nervous system is indicated. Vertebral-basilar insufficiency is, of course, most common in the population of patients over 50 years old (refer to Case Studies–8, p. 152).

b. Tumor

Pontine tumors, if localized to one side of the brainstem, cause contralateral hemiplegia and paralysis of the ipsilateral cranial nerves. These nerves are often interrupted in their intramedullary or intracranial course causing manifestations of peripheral nerve disease such as muscle weakness accompanied by atrophy. The Vth, VIth, VIIth or VIIIth nerves may be involved. If the tumors are intramedullary, dysconjugate eye movements and gaze nystagmus are common.

Cerebellar tumors give rise to different symptoms and signs depending upon the locus of the lesion. Gaze nystagmus and positional nystagmus may be observed with midline or paramidline tumors while hemisphere tumors usually produce defects limited to the limbs. Arteriovenous malformation may occur in the cerebellar midline or hemisphere and produces symptoms accordingly. If the tumor is calcified it may be noted on skull X-ray but the diagnosis is usually verified by angiography or pneumoencephalography.

c. Platybasia and other congenital abnormalities

In platybasia (basilar impression) pressure on the brainstem and cerebellar structures with compression of the basilar artery produces numerous symptoms and signs, among which gait disturbance and vertical nystagmus are characteristic. A congenital defect such as Arnold-Chiari malformation should also be considered in these cases.

d. Spino-cerebellar degeneration

Gaze nystagmus, positional nystagmus (direction-changing type), and positioning nystagmus (vertical type) are common. The characteristic findings of the optokinetic pattern test are demonstrated (refer to Case Studies–9, p. 154).

e. Multiple sclerosis

Multiple sclerosis may cause various ocular symptoms including gaze nystagmus, spontaneous or positional nystagmus (vertical or horizontal), and gaze palsy such as internuclear ophthalmoplegia long before the occurrence of other neurologic symptoms.

3. Cerebral Lesion

a. Tumor, abscess, meningitis
b. Epilepsy

Ablation of the temporal lobe due to tumor or abscess and inflammation in the subarachnoid space can produce vertigo or disturbance in equilibrium. Vertigo also occurs as an aura of epilepsy or as a seizure per se. In such cases it is necessary to examine the possibility of coexistence of peripheral and brainstem disorders.

VERTIGO AND DIZZINESS CAUSED BY HEAD INJURY

These cases can be divided into five groups (HOZAWA, 1961).

1. Group I

Peripheral vestibular disturbance is caused immediately by head injury. Labyrinthine fracture, labyrinthine hemorrhage or concussion belong to this group. In such cases the following symptoms are found: Hypoexcitability of the unilateral labyrinth is accompanied

by ipsilateral deafness.   Ispilateral facial palsy can often be observed.   Bleeding from
the ear is common.   Fracture of the labyrinth is confirmed by X-ray.

2.   Group II

The occurrence of peripheral vestibular disturbance is delayed some weeks to months
after head injury.   Ménièriform disorder or positional vertigo of the benign paroxysmal
type after head injury and the cervicovestibular syndrome due to traumatic spondylosis
deformans belong to this group.

3.   Group III

Neither central nor peripheral vestibular disturbance is confirmed by neuro-otological
examination, however the patient complains of dizziness or tinnitus.   In such cases,
neurosis or malingering may be suspected.

4.   Group IV

Central vestibular disturbance occurs without any evidence of accompanying cerebrospinal lesions.   In group IV the abnormalities can only be demonstrated by the neuro-
otological examination.

5.   Group V

Central vestibular disturbance is accompanied by other cerebrospinal symptoms.   Not
only neuro-otological but also other neurological examinations show pathological findings.
Utilizing X-ray tests (pneumoencephalography, angiography etc.) and electroencephalo-
graphy, abnormalities can often be observed.

MISCELLANEOUS

Since vertigo and dizziness encountered in other conditions such as polycythemia rubra
vera, sickle cell disease, diabetes mellitus, cardiovascular diseases, carotid sinus syndrome
etc. could be both central and peripheral vestibular disturbances, it is difficult to classify
them.

Recent Progress in Vestibular Research

Chapters on anatomy and physiology are not included in this book as our emphasis was
placed on the description of procedures and interpretation of the neuro-otological examination.   However, an attempt has been made to cover some recent advances concerning
the basic aspects of peripheral and central vestibular mechanisms.

The parts of the inner ear related to the equilibrium function of the body consist of the
three semicircular canals and the otolith organs, the utricle and the saccule.   The receptor
cells of the semicircular canals are stimulated by angular acceleration of the head, which
causes movement of the cupula endolymph system and leads to deflexion of the cupula and
of the sensory hairs.   The action of linear acceleration or gravity causes dislocation of the
otolithic membrane and the resultant bending of the sensory hairs stimulates the receptor
cells in the otolith organ.   However, the role played by the hair cell, the cupula or otolithic
membrane, and the endolymph in the process of such mechano-electric stimulus transduc-
tion is not entirely clear despite a number of recent investigations.

The cupula of the semicircular canals has been classically viewed as a swinging door
sitting in the ampulla.   Recent evidence suggests that this may not be so.   HILLMAN (1972)
reported that the cupula actually has a circumferential attachment to the ampullar wall

and thus forms a diaphragm across the ampulla. He envisioned that the cupula moves like a sail with its center having maximum motion. Compression of the semicircular canal beyond physiologic limits (such as could occur in head trauma) might result in detachment of the cupula at its apex, a kind of safety valve mechanism. The cupula could then assume the classical swinging door appearance. OMAN and YOUNG (1972) in a theoretical consideration of the motion of the cupula find that the pressure gradients across the ampulla resulting from angular acceleration would result in extremely minute deviations of the cupula. Thus gross swinging door type motion would be unneccessary to explain the physiologic range of cupular motion.

Ultrastructural observation of the vestibular sensory epithelia of mammals and birds has demonstrated two types of sensory cells, i.e. the flask-shaped type I cells and the cylindrical type II cells (WERSÄLL, 1956). These cells have a marked difference in their contacts with afferent nerve endings; large chalices are formed around type I cells and smaller club endings are formed in the synaptic region of type II cells. In addition to afferent fibers the vestibular labyrinth is innervated by efferent fibers (PETROFF, 1955; WERSÄLL, 1956; ENGSTRÖM, 1958; GACEK, 1960). The connection of the efferent fibers to the receptor cells is also different for the type I and II cells. The efferent fibers can be demonstrated at the level of the brainstem (ROSS and CORTESINA, 1965). Thus the existence of a closed feedback loop between the labyrinthine receptors and the vestibular nuclei or reticular formation has been suggested.

The sensory hairs on the outer surface of the hair cells are divided into the kinocilium and the stereocilia. The kinocilium located in the periphery of the hair bundle is the longest and the stereocilia are arranged in order of decreasing height away from the kinocilium. Such an asymmetric arrangement of the hair bundle on each cell surface has suggested a characteristic organization in each sensory area of the labyrinth (LOWENSTEIN and WERSÄLL, 1959). For example, the kinocilium in the cristae of the lateral semicircular canal is regularly found on the utricular side, and in the cristae of the vertical canals on the opposite side. This may be related to the difference in directional sensitivity of the cupular movement between the lateral and the vertical (anterior and posterior) canals. However, functional significance of the detailed structures including that of the efferent system is still not clear.

Recently HILLMAN (1969, 1972) has proposed a mechanism to explain how motion of the labrinthine cilia can result in a modulation of vestibular nerve activity. The stereocilia which stand on a rigid cuticular plate cannot move vertically but are free to slide at their distal ends. The single kinocilium however stands over a notch in the cuticular plate but is attached to the stereocilia by filamentous processes at its distal end. Thus, when a force is directed toward the kinociliary end of the hair cell a plunging motion results in producing an inward deformation of the cell membrane at the kinociliary base. A force in the opposite direction would result in an outward rounding of the membrane. This deformation of the notch membrane could produce the conductance changes which are thought to modulate the transmitter release and modify VIIIth nerve activity.

Vestibular impulses from the labyrinthine receptors reach the vestibular nuclei and are transmitted to various portions of the nervous system such as the eye muscle motor nuclei, the spinal cord, the cerebellum, and the reticular formation. On the other hand, numerous afferent projections from other parts of the central nervous system converge onto the vestibular nuclei. Thus it is certain that the vestibular nuclei act not only as a single relay station but rather as an integrator of the activities from the periphery and from other sensory structures.

The anatomical and functional organization of the vestibular nuclei consists of four main divisions, the superior, the lateral, the medial and the descending (or inferior) nuclei. Of particular interest is the demonstration of a somatotopic organization within the lateral vestibular nucleus (BRODAL et al., 1962). The lateral nucleus is divided into a "neck and forelimb region", a "trunk region", and a "hindlimb region" according to the terminal sites in the spinal cord of the nerve fibers originating from the nucleus; the fibers to the cervical cord arise from the rostroventral part of the nucleus and those to the lumbosacral cord from its dorsocaudal part. Moreover, the primary vestibular fibers are restricted to the forelimb region and the afferent fibers from the spinal cord as well as from the anterior vermis of the cerebellum reach mainly the hindlimb region. In addition to this vestibulo-spinal connection it was found that another pathway, though relatively modest, arises from the medial vestibular nucleus and ends at the midthoracic levels (NYBERG-HANSEN, 1964). The latter is called the medial vestibulospinal tract in contrast to the lateral vestibulospinal tract. Similar structural organization was also noted within the other vestibular nuclei (BRODAL et al., 1962).

Electrophysiological studies have confirmed the somatotopic organization of the vestibular nuclei suggested by anatomical studies and, furthermore, have afforded new data concerning the functional aspects of the nuclei. The identification of different types of second vestibular neurons (GERNANDT, 1949; DUENSING and SCHAEFER, 1958) has now been established. The majority of the second order neurons responding to stimulation of the lateral semicircular canal increase their frequency of discharge during ipsilateral acceleration, i.e. clockwise rotation for the right labyrinth, and decrease their discharge frequency during contralateral acceleration. This pattern of responses, called the type I response, is similar to that of the primary afferent fibers in the lateral semicircular canal (LOWENSTEIN and SAND, 1940). Finally, four types of response of the second order vestibular neurons were described by DUENSING and SCHAEFER, and further details of their characteristics have been studied (SHIMAZU and PRECHT, 1965; PRECHT and SHIMAZU, 1965; WILSON et al., 1967).

Recently the existence and nature of the commissural fibers between the vestibular nuclei of each side was confirmed physiologically (SHIMAZU and PRECHT, 1966; WILSON et al., 1968) and anatomically (LADPLI and BRODAL, 1968). From these studies it was concluded that the crossed inhibitory influence is mediated from the contralateral to the ipsilateral vestibular nuclei via the commissural fibers and not via vestibulo-reticular loops. This mutual interaction may serve for producing highly sensitive outputs from the vestibular nuclei.

Among the various outputs from the vestibular nuclei the vestibulo-ocular projection has been extensively studied, both clinically and physiologically. The semicircular canals and the otolith organs, at least the utricle, exert precise and powerful control over the extraocular muscles (SZENTAGOTHAI, 1950; COHEN et al., 1964; SUZUKI et al., 1969). Anatomical studies have shown that the primary afferent fibers from the semicircular canals and the otolith organs terminate in portions of the vestibular nuclei which are largely separate from each other (STEIN and CARPENTER, 1967; GACEK, 1969). The semicircular canals send axons mainly to the rostral portions of the vestibular nuclei and the otolith organs project axons primarily to their rather caudal portions. The rostral projections from the individual vestibular nuclei are specifically distributed in the eye muscle motor nuclei via the ipsilateral or contralateral medial longitudinal fasciculus, although there is still some controversy on these projections (McMASTERS et al., 1966; TARLOV, 1970; GACEK, 1971). The abducens and trochlear nuclei innervate the ipsilateral external rectus and the contralateral superior oblique muscles respectively, while the oculomotor nuclei have a clear cut somatotopical organization of motoneurons projecting to the other extraocular muscles (WARWICK, 1953; TARLOV and TARLOV, 1971). These results strongly suggest that there must be closely related connections between the primary vestibular fibers coming from individual receptor organs and the motoneurons of the eye muscle motor nuclei innervating different extraocular muscles. There are still some discrepancies between the anatomical and physiological findings but some of the major aspects of the vestibulo-ocular reflex arc have been established. The same may be said of problems on the vestibulo-reticular and the vestibulo-cerebellar interactions, which are important in the modulation or production of semicircular canal-ocular and otolith-ocular reflexes (for reviews see COHEN, 1971).

Recent physiological studies have shown the nature of the cerebello-vestibular interactions; the Purkinje cells of the cerebellar vermis exert corticofugal inhibition onto neurons in the vestibular nuclei (ITO and YOSHIDA, 1964). This is contrary to the excitatory action of the cerebellar nuclei upon their target cells (ITO et al., 1970). Moreover, the influence of the superior vestibular nucleus has been shown to be purely inhibitory to the eye muscle motor nuclei (HIGHSTEIN and ITO, 1971). Oculomotor effects following stimulation and destruction of the superior vestibular nucleus can be explained by the anatomical evidence of fiber connection and the inhibitory nature of the cells in the superior vestibular nucleus (UEMURA and COHEN, 1972, 1973).

In brief, research within the vestibular system in progress during the past decade has been focussed on identifying the structural and functional units in each portion of this system and, further, on clarifying their characteristics in detail. Consequently, certain aspects of the vestibular mechanism have become clarified. On the other hand, many complex facets of the system remain unclear and even complicate the interpretation of clinical symptoms and signs. However, it is certain that continuing research is bringing us closer to a complete understanding of the vestibular system. Furthermore, BRODAL (1969, p. 687) commenting on this stated "an understanding of the complexities in the organization of the nervous system will relieve the neurologist of the 'moral obligation' to make his findings fit preconceived traditional conceptions". These circumstances may afford us a reason to write a new book on the neuro-otological examination without undue emphasis on the past history of development of this subject.

II

History-Taking

In neuro-otology as in all branches of medicine, a good clinical history can hold the key to a correct diagnosis. The patient's complaint should be carefully documented from the onset of the illness. Sometimes the examiner tries to record the complaints using technical terms. This can lead to inaccurate histories and wrong diagnoses since the patient often attaches his own meaning to the particular technical words which he employs. It is important that the patient is asked to describe the complaints in his own words but the meaning of the history must be clarified by the examiner who should gently lead the history along the proper lines to accurately characterize the illness.

History of the Present Illness

VERTIGO AND DIZZINESS

CHARACTER AND SEVERITY—What is the nature of the complaint?

Initially it is the best to have the patient express his complaint in his own words. There is a wide variation in what a patient means by "dizziness". The complaint of dizziness can be divided into four groups from the view point of diagnostic significance.

(1) A turning sensation of the body or surroundings.
(2) A swaying or floating sensation of the body laterally, back- and forward or up- and downward.
(3) Disequilibrium such as a falling tendency.
(4) Miscellaneous; lightheadedness, blacking out, fainting and others.

(1) and (2) A turning or swaying sensation:
The term vertigo is defined, for example, as "consciousness of disordered orientation regarding the body in space" (BRAIN, 1938) or "hallucination (experience of sensation without external stimulation) of movement" (JONGKEES, 1953; CAWTHORNE, 1964). The latter definition is preferable because it is expressed in a more definite form. The "hallucination" of vertigo is usually accompanied by the recognition that it is a false sensation of movement. According to this definition, the sensations of turning and swaying may be included in true vertigo.

Unilateral acute disorders of the vestibular system may cause a turning sensation. The vestibular system contains the peripheral labyrinth, vestibular nerve, vestibular nuclei and higher vestibular pathways including the cerebral cortex. Because dysfunction at any level may cause a turning sensation it is difficult to attach significance for topical diagnosis to this symptom. A swaying sensation may originate from a unilateral subacute or bilateral (either acute or subacute) disorder of the vestibular system, but the location of the pathology responsible for this sensation is often obscure just as with a turning sensation. These sensations often overlap and may be caused by the same locus of dysfunction, i.e. the turning sensation experienced at the acute episode of Ménière's disease is often commuted to a swaying sensation which may linger on for weeks after the acute episode is over.

Vertigo is usually accompanied by an autonomic disturbance such as nausea, vomiting, cold sweating and diarrhea. The severity of these varies among individuals; however, primary disease of the digestive system should be suspected in an extreme case.

(3) Disequilibrium such as a falling tendency:

The complaint of a falling tendency may indicate recognition of disequilibrium. When the vestibular system on one side is slowly losing its activity as in the case of an acoustic tumor, the patient recognizes only disequilibruim and is not disturbed by vertigo. On the other hand, a patient with an acute labyrinthine disorder is usually disturbed by vertigo and disequilibrium. This is a helpful point in differential diagnosis.

In summary, the character of the complaint caused by unilateral disorders of the vestibular system may vary from a sensation of turning to that of swaying depending upon the abruptness of the underlying process. When the process is extremely slow, disequilibrium of the body is the only perceptible symptom.

(4) Miscellaneous; lightheadedness, blacking out, fainting and others:

Miscellaneous complaints may originate from diseases not related to the labyrinth, such as hypertension, hypotension, carotid sinus syndrome, epilepsy, etc. Drop attacks with quadriplegia usually without loss of consciousness, which occur after hyperextension or rotation of the neck, are suggestive of vertebral-basilar insufficiency.

PRECIPITATING FACTORS—*What was the patient doing just before vertigo began?*

Factors which may precipitate an episode in either a direct or an indirect fashion should be considered. It is frequently found that episodes of Ménière's disease begin after a period of stress and that vestibular neuronitis is preceded by an infection of the upper respiratory tract. Furthermore, whether the assumption of a specific posture preceded the attack may provide important information for diagnosis. Although an episode of Ménière's disease may appear suddenly without any apparent relation to the head position, the so-called positional vertigo (or nystagmus) of the benign paroxysmal type is induced by assuming a critical head position. In such cases, vertigo often appears with a latency of about 5 seconds after assuming this critical position and recedes or disappears within 30 seconds even if the same position is maintained. Subsequently, reassuming this position is less effective in evoking vertigo. Any position of the body aggravating or lessening the symptom during the episode should be described. These descriptions are valuable in terms of examining positional or positioning nystagmus. Cervical vertigo (RYAN and COPE, 1955) and vertigo due to basilar insufficiency (DENNY-BROWN, 1953) are provoked by the position of the head relative to the body, but not by the head position itself. Also, in Bruns' symptom (BRUNS, 1902; ALPERS and YASKIN, 1944) caused by fourth ventricle tumors, the attack of vertigo, headache, vomiting and poor vision is often provoked by a change in head position.

THE MODE OF ONSET AND SUBSEQUENT COURSE—*How did the symptom begin and how does it vary?*

Although an attack of Ménière's disease may arise suddenly and largely subside within hours, vertigo due to labyrinthitis secondary to otitis media often remains rather persistent-

ly.   If the vertiginous attack is recurrent, the variation in frequency and severity should
be recorded.   WILLIAMS (1965) noted that the attacks of Ménière's disease tend to come
in groups or clusters.

AUDITORY SYMPTOMS

It is necessary to document historically whether the symptoms of hearing loss and tinnitus
are related to a concomitant vertiginous attack because the auditory symptoms in Ménière's disease sometimes precede the vertiginous attack by years.   In such cases, for example, tinnitus may become accentuated or vary in nature during the attack.

From the relationship between the course of deafness and the onset of vertigo, Lermoyez's
syndrome which consists of sudden restoration of hearing during episodic attacks of vertigo
was differentiated from Ménière's disease (LERMOYEZ, 1919).   However, since the underlying process seems similar to, if not identical with, that present in the ordinary case of
Ménière's disease, Lermoyez's syndrome should be considered a variety of Ménière's
disease (WILLIAMS, 1952; ALTMAN, 1955; STOECKLIN, 1957; GOLDING-WOOD, 1960).

The absence of the complaint of deafness does not rule out a hearing loss.   For example,
the patient is sometimes unaware of the occurrence of complete deafness in one ear during
an attack of vertigo.   Furthermore, the presence of hearing loss limited to the high frequency range is often only detected by a hearing test.

Other auditory symptoms are diplacusis (distortion in pitch), and the phenomenon of
recruitment (distortion of loudness), which is recognized by the patient's complaint that
loud noises bother him.   These phenomena are indicative of the presence of inner ear
deafness and particularly of Ménière's disease.   A sensation of fullness in the ear is one
of the most consistent findings in Ménière's disease.   Thus, when adding this symptom
to vertigo, hearing loss and tinnitus, ALFARO (1958) proposed that these four symptoms
should constitute the tetrad of Ménière's disease.

SYMPTOMS NOT RELATED TO THE STATOACOUSTIC NERVE

It is an important problem to separate diseases involving the central nervous system
from those involving the inner ear.   Certain symptoms, such as blurred vision, motor or
sensory disturbances and loss of consciousness, which may accompany vertigo strongly suggest
that the cause of the vertigo is present in the central nervous (or cardiovascular) system.
Among intracranial diseases vertebral-basilar insufficiency may be the most common cause
of vertigo and must be noted particularly as a warning of occlusive vascular disease.   Such
patients rarely have auditory symptoms, but often have other symptoms, such as aberration
in vision, numbness around the mouth, somatic motor and sensory disturbances on one or
both sides, difficulty in phonation and swallowing, or other brainstem signs.   On the
other hand, there is the possibility that, if circulatory disturbance due to arteriosclerosis is
limited to the labyrinthine artery, a reverse combination of symptoms, i.e. the presence of
auditory symptoms and the absence of other neurological symptoms, may occnr.   When
symptoms and signs related to basilar artery insufficiency are produced by exercise of the
upper limb, the subclavian steal syndrome (brachial-basilar insufficiency syndrome) resulting from proximal occlusion of the subclavian artery should be suspected (NORTH et al.,
1962).

Ocular symptoms may occur concomitantly with vestibulo-auditory symptoms in Cogan's
syndrome, i.e. nonsyphilitic keratitis with vestibulo-auditory symptoms (COGAN, 1945;
STEVENS, 1954), Vogt-Koyanagi-Harada syndrome (uveomeningoencephalic syndrome)
and also in sympathetic ophthalmia.

Congenital nystagmus usually is not accompanied by the complaint of oscillopsia, i.e. an optic illusory movement of a viewed stationary object, although patients with acquired fixation nystagmus may complain of this difficulty. Similar complaints may be noticed in cases of bilateral or severe unilateral involvement of the vestibular system, but in such cases oscillopsia is predominantly recognized during walking or sudden head movements.

The general impression which the patient affords during the taking of the history is often useful for diagnosis. For example, the examiner should carefully evaluate the severity of the patient's anxiety and depression. The examiner should also differentiate between the stress which provokes the episode and the anxiety reaction which results from the episode. In order to estimate emotional factors objectively, the Cornell Medical Index (C.M.I.), a simple scoring method available for psychological screening, is useful (BRODMAN et al., 1949; FUKAMACHI, 1959).

Past Medical History and Family History

In the approach to the patient with vertigo, one should ask about a past history of otitis media, ear surgery, head or acoustic trauma, use of certain drugs having an ototoxic action, and syphilis. When the patient is suspected of congenital nystagmus, an inquiry about the presence of nystagmus during childhood is essential, and when visual disturbances including nystagmus are present in other members of the family, a hereditary factor may be suggested. On the other hand, since the occurrence of nystagmus in specific occupations, such as miners and train dispatchers, has been described, the occupation of the patient should be a part of every medical history.

III

Methods of the Neuro-Otological Examination

The Neurologic Examination

The purpose of this chapter is to present the essential features of the neurologic examination and to discuss the differential diagnosis of various symptoms and signs. Special emphasis will be given to clinical entities which lie between neurology and otology, as it is sometimes difficult to distinguish in which domain the pathology lies. The otologist is not infrequently consulted by a patient with signs or symptoms which may seem related to the labyrinth but which are caused by dysfunction of the central or peripheral nervous system. The ability to perform a neurologic examination and roughly localize the area of difficulty will speed the patient towards proper treatment.

The neurological examination begins with the history. Effort should be made to obtain spontaneous complaints before any specific or leading questions are asked. By listening carefully to the patient's complaints the examiner can often be directed to a particular area of dysfunction within the nervous system. Then the examiner may ask more specific questions. The date of onset of symptoms, progress or remission of complaints and history of past illness should be elicited. A reliable history will often suggest the diagnosis. For example, though the complaint, perhaps of dizziness, may seem related to acute labyrinthine dysfunction, a previous history of blurred or double vision, vertigo, dizziness, slurred speech or numbness around the face may indicate lesions of the vertebral-basilar arterial system. The dissemination in time or location of neurologic complaints which point to involvement of several areas of the nervous system signify multiple sclerosis in a younger patient. Thus, the importance of the neurologic history cannot be overemphasized.

If neurological disease is suspected a complete routine neurological examination should be performed, including examination of the mental status, the cranial nerves, the motor and the sensory systems.

The examination may be divided as follows:
1. Mental status examination
2. Cranial nerve examination
3. Motor examination including tests of coordination
4. Sensory examination

MENTAL STATUS EXAMINATION

Every patient should be given a mental status examination as abnormal mental processes are one indicator of cerebral dysfunction. Also if the mental status of the patient is in doubt any history previously obtained from the patient must obviously be re-evaluated. The examination may be divided into the following categories:

(1) Level of Alertness: Is the patient fully awake and alert or is he drowsy, stuporous

or comatose? Can the patient be roused to a state of full alertness? If the patient is less than fully awake and alert some degree of cerebral dysfunction may be implied.

(2) Orientation: The patient should be able to state his name, age, the year, month and day of the week. He should have a rough idea of the time of day and should probably know the examiner's name especially if previously introduced.

(3) General information: The patient should be familiar with matters of common knowledge, such as the name of the president or prime minister of his country, and the mayor of his city or town.

(4) Memory: Recent and past memory should be tested.

(5) Naming of objects and body parts: The examiner may point to the patient's hand or other body part and ask the patient to name it. Objects such as a pencil or pen may also be used as test objects to be named.

(6) Right-left orientation and mimicry: The patient is asked to touch his left ear with his right hand. He is then instructed to mimic the examiner's movements such as touching the left ear with the left hand, touching the nose with the index finger, etc.

(7) Simple calculation, spelling, reading: The patient is asked to spell 3, 4, or 5 letter words; simple calculations are also tested. He is also requested to read aloud the headline of a newspaper.

(8) Reversals: The patient is asked to reverse the spelling of 3, 4 or 5 letter words, and to count backwards from 20 to 1, the inability to reverse spelling and counting are reliable indicators of mental dysfunction.

Although a more complete evaluation of the various functions of language is possible (a complete aphasic status), the ability to successfully perform the screening mental status examination (especially 5, 6, 7, and 8) may be taken as an indication of normalcy. If difficulty with language is present, this indicates cerebral dysfunction of the dominant hemisphere.

CRANIAL NERVE EXAMINATION

The cranial nerves may be listed as follows.

	NERVE	FUNCTION
CN I	Olfactory nerve	Smell
CN II	Optic nerve	Vision
CN III	Oculomotor nerve	Pupil motor, eye movement, eye lid motor
CN IV	Trochlear nerve	Eye movement
CN V	Trigeminal nerve	Facial sensation, jaw movement
CN VI	Abducens nerve	Eye movement
CN VII	Facial nerve	Facial movement, taste anterior 2/3 of tongue, stapedius motor
CN VIII	Stato-acoustic nerve	Hearing, vestibular function
CN IX	Glossopharyngeus nerve	Pharynx motor, pharynx sensation, taste posterior 1/3 of tongue
CN X	Vagus nerve	Pharynx, larynx, motor autonomic
CN XI	Spinal accessory nerve	Motor to sternomastoid and trapezius
CN XII	Hypoglossal nerve	Motor nerve of the tongue

CN I Examination of Olfaction

A small vial of some pungent substance, such as cloves or other spices are often used to test smell. The vial should be exposed to each nostril in succession. Loss of smell may be unilateral, bilateral, complete or partial.   It has been stated that complete loss of smell is associated with impairment of taste, but this is not invariably so.

Olfactory dysfunction may be caused by a compression of the olfactory tracts by meningioma, metastatic or primary neoplasm, aneurism or other space occupying lesion of the anterior fossa.   Olfactory hallucinations may occur with temporal lobe seizures, or a strong odor, usually unpleasant, may be the aura of grand mal epilepsy, but in these cases the sense of smell is usually unimpaired.

The diagnostic value of loss of the sense of smell is seen mainly when this defect is part of a symptom complex rather than an isolated finding.

CN II   Examination of Vision

Impairment of vision may originate from a disturbance of function of the cornea, lens, optic media, retina, optic nerve, chiasm, optic tract, central optic pathways or the visual cortex.   Often a disturbance of eye movement or vestibular function will cause some difficulty in vision as well.   Visual dysfunction may be an isolated phenomenon, as in the case of lesions of the retina or optic nerve or it may occur as part of a symptom complex. Occasionally the patient may be unaware of a visual dysfunction which is revealed by the examination.

At first, the patient should be carefully observed.   Does he seem to pay equal attention to both the right and left fields of vision or does he neglect objects on one side or the other? If so, a homonomous hemianopia or a complete hemispacial syndrome may be present. Homonomous hemianopia is a loss of vision in the homonomous hemifields of vision of both eyes, and is theoretically caused by unilateral lesions in the visual pathway at any point central to the optic chiasm, but is in practice almost always associated with disease of the posterior two thirds of the opposite cerebral hemisphcre.   Homonomous hemianopia may not be accompanied by other signs of cerebral dysfunction.

Gross impairment of vision:

In examining visual function, each eye should be individually tested.   The subject should be seated opposite the examiner in a well lighted room, and should be instructed to cover one eye with his hand.   The subject is then instructed to look at the examiner's nose and not to further move his eyes.   The examiner then begins by bringing his hand from beyond the periphery of the subject's visual field towards the center asking the subject to report when he sees the hand (see Fig. 1a).   This procedure is then repeated from the other side, as well as from above and below in order to test all four quadrants of the visual field.   This is a gross testing method designed to bring out severe visual field defects, such as hemifield defects or large scotomas.   The visual fields when tested by this method should extend 180° in all directions, being limited on the nasal side by the height of the bridge of the nose.   It is often helpful for the examiner to compare his own visual field to the patient's.   Sitting directly opposite the patient and looking at the patient's eye with the examiner's opposite eye, i.e. the patient's right eye, examiner's left—if the hand is brought into play equidistant between the patient and the examiner, the examiner's visual field may be simultaneously observed and compared to that of the patient.

More subtle defects in vision:

Other tests of vision.

(1)   The red match test* of visual function.   This is a simple and sensitive test of vision. The underlying principle of this test is that the visual fields for color are smaller in area

---

* This test was introduced by Dr. M.B. Bender, Head of the Neurology Service of the Mt. Sinai School of Medicine, and has been successfully performed at the bedside or in the office by graduates of that department for many years.

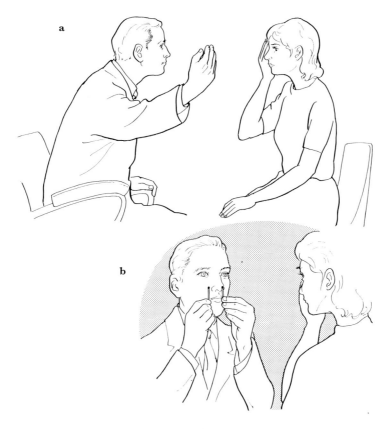

Fig. 1

a: Gross examination of the visual fields by hand confrontation. The patient looks at the examiner's right eye with her left eye. Her right eye is covered. The examiner moves his hand from beyond the periphery of the patient's field of vision toward the center of the field. The patient is asked to report when she first sees the hand. Further explanation is in the text.

b: The red match test. The patient covers one eye and is asked to look at the match placed on the examiner's nose. A second match is placed on the examiner's cheek. The patient is asked to compare the color of the two matches.

than those for white or black and also that progressive visual dysfunction of almost any etiology affects color perception before it affects form or motion perception.

The examiner faces the patient as previously stated; each eye is again individually tested. As shown in Fig. 1b, the examiner places one match on the tip of his nose and a second match on his cheek. The patient is asked to report upon the color of both matches, i.e. are they the same, or is one or the other pale or white. If one match is perceived as pale or white, a defect in the visual field subtended is indicated.

In cases of central scotoma the match displayed on the nose may or may not be perceived, but if seen the color will be reported to be white or pale by comparison to the lateral match. It can be appreciated that by moving the position of the second match all four fields of vision may be investigated.

    (2)   Double simultaneous stimulation
    (3)   Use of pseudoisochromatic plates
    (4)   Determination of localization within the visual space
    (5)   Visual acuity

For a complete description of these and other tests of visual function see BENDER (1967), KESTEN-
BAUM (1961).

Perimetry:

Perimetric examination is of course unsurpassed for accurately localizing small visual
field defects. It is also useful for accurately following the course of progressive defects,
such as gradually enlarging bitemporal field loss resulting from pressure on the chiasm
secondary to a pituitary adenoma, an enlarging third ventricle, or other space occupying
lesions in the chiasmal region.

Odd shaped monocular scotomas, ring or sector defects or other unusual field losses may
be due to disease of the lens or ocular media and should be referred to the ophthalmologist.

Fundoscopy:

The retina and optic disc should be examined with an ophthalmoscope as the retina is
the only place in the body where a direct view of the vascular bed is readily visible to the
physician. Abnormalities of the retina can give valuable information about systemic
diseases, and signs of increased intracranial pressure may indicate intracranial pathology.
A pathologic appearance of the retina and optic disc often is correlated with the findings of
the visual field examination. For example, choked discs, often seen with increased intracranial pressure, may be correlated with enlarged blind spots and suggest that this part
of the visual examination should be carried out more carefully. The appearance of the
vascular bed may suggest systemic disease such as generalized vascular disease, and rarely
tumor exudates such as Hodgkin's exudates may be seen.

Lastly, the nerve head may appear swollen in cases of optic neuritis correlated with
central scotoma and will appear shrunken and white late in the course of this illness.

CN III, IV, VI   Examination of Eye Movement

The examination of eye movement encompasses the examination of the function of the
IIIrd, IVth and VIth cranial nerves; however, abnormal eye movements may also be
present in visual or vestibular as well as primary eye muscle dysfunction.

The third cranial nerve has four branches which innervate four different extra-ocular
muscles; the superior rectus which elevates the eye, the medial rectus which moves the
eye medially, the inferior rectus which depresses the eye, and the inferior oblique which
elevates and rotates the globe. There are also fibers to the levator palpebrae muscle which
elevates the lid and to the pupillary construction muscles innervated by the Edinger-
Westphal nucleus. The ciliary muscle which controls the thickness of the lens is also
innervated by the IIIrd nerve.

The trochlear nerve innervates the superior oblique muscle which depresses and intorts
the eye. Fourth nerve action is difficult to distinguish in the presence of a normal third
nerve, but with paralysis of the IIIrd nerve, such as occurs in peripheral diabetic neuropathy, pure IVth nerve action may be seen. The VIth or abducens nerve innervates the
lateral rectus muscle which deviates the eye laterally.

The trochlear nerve and the superior rectus branch of the IIIrd nerve cross to innervate
the contralateral eye muscles; the nerves to the medial rectus, inferior rectus, inferior
oblique and lateral rectus muscles are uncrossed.

The examination of eye movements begins with observation of the patient. Normally
the eyes should be in conjugate positions in the orbits, palpebral fissures should be of equal
size and there should be no spontaneous nystagmus. Normal eye movements should be
conjugate in all cases. (Convergence movements are of course an exception to this.) The
patient is asked to look to the right, to the left, up, and down. These movements should
be accomplished easily and smoothly. Some head movement may be brought into play

by those commands but the eye movement should always precede the head movement by a fraction of a second.

Pursuit: Next the patient is asked to follow the examiner's finger as it moves from left to right and up to down. This maneuver should bring the eyes to the extremes of the orbits. Cogwheeling or jerky eye movements may be elicited in Parkinson's disease. These should be differentiated from nystagmus. A few beats of end or terminal nystagmus as the eyes move to the extremes of the orbits are considered within normal limits.

Oculo-cephalic reflex:

The oculo-cephalic reflex is then tested. As shown in Fig. 2, the patient is asked to look at the examiner and his head is passively moved from side to side and up and down. Nomally the eyes deviate in the direction opposite to passive head movement and then recenter.

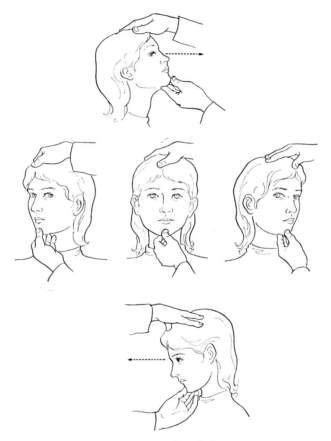

Fig. 2 The oculocephalic test.
The test begins with the head facing forward and the eyes centered (center drawing). The patient is instructed to look at the examiner who remains directly in front of her. The examiner then grasps the patient's head and moves it right and left, up and down noting the position of the eyes at each new head position. The arrows in the top and bottom figures indicate the direction of gaze.

If a gaze palsy or paresis is present, eye movements may be elicited by various testing methods. The most compelling eye movements are produced by instructing the patient to fixate his eyes on the examiner and then moving his head from side to side or up and down, instructing the patient to follow a moving finger or object is the next most compelling procedure and finally, eye movements performed on command are the least compelling.

Failure of conjugate deviation in a lateral direction indicates a gaze deficit as may be found in cerebral or brain stem disease. A paralysis of vertical movements indicates bilateral brain stem disease while a unilateral paralysis of eye movement in a given direction usually indicates peripheral nerve dysfunction. As a general rule, acute cerebral dysfunction causes a paralysis of conjugate gaze to the side opposite to the lesion, while brain stem dysfunction causes gaze paralysis to the side of the lesion.

Internuclear ophthalmoplegia is a condition in which horizontal eye movements are dysconjugate. It is caused by a disruption of the fibers travelling in the medial longitudinal fasciculus (MLF) of the brain stem. The medial rectus muscle on the side of the lesion fails to contract during pursuit or on command; however, ocular convergence is preserved. Thus, with left sided MLF damage when the patient looks to the right the left eye remains in the midline while the right eye deviates laterally and has nystagmus. Unilateral internuclear ophthalmoplegia is often present transiently early in the course of vascular disease of the brain while bilateral internuclear ophthalmoplegia is most commonly caused by multiple sclerosis.

Convergence:

Ocular convergence is tested by instructing the patient to look at a distant object and then at a near object. As mentioned, convergence is preserved in internuclear ophthalmoplegia.

Optokinetic Nystagmus: Optokinetic nystagmus may easily be elicited by having the patient read the numbers on a tape measure moved slowly from side to side or up to down about twelve inches in front of his eyes. This nystagmus should be present in all directions, and of equal magnitude and intensity in opposite directions.

Optokinetic nystagmus may be valuable in the localization of brain dysfunction (refer to the chapter of OKN).*

Pupillary reactions: Normal pupils are round, regular and equal. The pupils of both eyes should constrict briskly when a strong light is shone into either eye. If both pupils react to light shone into one eye but do not react to light in the other eye this indicates blindness in the eye which caused no reaction. Pupillary reactions should also be tested for accomodative changes. When the patient fixates a distinct object the pupils should dilate, but fixation on a near object should be accompanied by pupillary constriction. Ocular convergence and blinking are also accompaneid by pupillary constriction.

CN V   Examination of Facial Sensation and Jaw Movement

The trigeminal nerve supplies sensation over the face and part of the scalp. It also controls jaw movements. The sensory area supplied by this nerve is divided into the ophthalmic, mandibular and maxillary areas. All modalities of sensation should be tested in all three divisions of the trigeminal nerve distribution bilaterally. The patient is asked to discriminate between the touch of a finger and a pinprick as well as between hot and cold. Sensitivity to vibration is also tested. The afferent limb of the corneal reflex is tested by blowing on the cornea. This stimulation elicits a blink which should be bilateral.

Both jaw opening and closure should be tested. If there is some involvement of the motor divison of the Vth nerve the jaw deviates toward the affected side on opening. If the involvement has been present for some time, there may be asymmetry in the temporal fossa due to temporalis muscle wasting.

Dysfunction of the Vth nerve may be caused by compression of the nerve external to the skull by a tumor such as a neurofibroma or by metastatic lesions. The nerve may

---

* For a complete description of its use see also KESTENBAUM, A.: Methods of Neuro-Ophthalmologic Examination. Grune and Stratton, 1960.

also be damaged by tumor growth inside the skull, such as an acoustic neurinoma. Glioma of the brain stem and vascular disease of the brain stem may damage the nerve or nucleus within the brain stem.

Tic doloreaux is a symptom complex of extremely severe bright episodic pains in the face along the distribution of any or all of the sensory branches of the Vth nerve. The episdoes are sudden in onset and may be triggered by jaw movement or by touching a particular area of the face (trigger zone). The paroxysmal nature of these pains has been likened to a seizure discharge and this view has gained support clinically as an attack may be terminated by intravenous administration of anticonvulsants. The successful long term treatment of this condition with anticonvulsants also supports this thesis.

There are various conditions that can produce pain in the face, such as infected sinuses or carious teeth, but the characteristic history of trigeminal neuralgia should make the distinction between this and any other conditions clear.

CN VII   Examination of Facial Movement, Taste

The facial nerve is the motor nerve to the face and innervates the taste receptors on the anterior two-thirds of the tongue. The patient should be observed for facial asymmetries, i.e. is one palpebral fissure wider than the other or does one side of the mouth droop? Are the nasolabial folds equal in size? The facial innervation of the forehead receives bilateral cerebral upper motor neuron control while that of the lower two thirds of the face, including the orbicularis oculi, is only controlled by the contralateral cerebral hemisphere. Thus in a peripheral lesion such as Bell's palsy the whole side of the face is involved, while a unilateral lesion of the cerebrum such as can occur in vascular disease usually spares the forehead.

Eyelid closure is tested by asking the patient to shut his eyes while the examiner manually tries to open them. (It is noted that the eyeball normally rolls up during eye closure. Movement of the globe in another direction may indicate faulty reinnervation of the eye muscles secondary to a peripheral IIIrd nerve lesion such as diabetic neuropathy or may indicate unilateral dysfunction of the oculomotor system at the level of the cerebrum.) The orbicularis oris is tested by forcibly trying to open the patient's lips while the patient keeps them tightly pressed together. Lastly the platysma muscles should be tested by asking the patient to strongly turn down the corners of his mouth; these muscles then usually contract. If the neck is flexed against the resistance of the examiner's hand the platysma muscles may also become active. Hyperacusis is a common symptom in Bell's palsy. This is thought to be due to malfunction of the stapedius muscle, secondary to the disease of the VIIth nerve.

Taste should be tested by first drying the protruded tongue and then placing a drop of salt solution, sugar solution or a bitter substance such as quinine on the tongue and asking the patient to report the taste. The anterior two-thirds and posterior one-third of the tongue should be examined differentially as their innervation is different.

Lesions of the facial nerve may be caused by the same range of process as affects the Vth nerve.

CN VIII   Examination of Hearing, Balance, and Vestibular Reactions

The stato-acoustic nerve is the subject of another chapter but in addition the performance of double simultaneous caloric examination will now be described. As stated, the caloric test mainly affects the horizontal and anterior semicircular canals, the posterior canal being largely unaffected. Water 10°F above or below the body temperature should be used. If the head is in an upright position the effects of thermal stimulation upon the vertical canals will be the ones primarily manifested.   Any component of horizontal canal action will be diminished by bilateral simultaneous irrigation while vertical canal action will be additive.   Double simultaneous cold stimulation will produce upward nystagmus; the patient may fall forward if asked to stand.   Hot stimulation will produce downward nystagmus, and backward falling.

Bilateral caloric tests are helpful in the evaluation of vertical eye movement disorders such as occur with lesions of the pretectum or in bilateral brain stem disease.

CN IX, X   Examination of the Pharynx Motor, Pharyngeal Sensation and Taste

Taste on the posterior one-third of the tongue is routinely tested.   The gag reflex should be tested bilaterally, by touching the back of the throat with a cotton swab.   Swallowing should be tested by observing the patient drink.

The uvula should be in the midline position and upon phonation the palate should elevate equally bilaterally.   The quality of the voice should be observed for hoarseness.

The IXth, Xth, XIth and XIIth nerves may be involved internally or externally at their exit from the base of the skull, internally within the skull or within the brain stem in their intramedullary course.

CN XI   Examination of the Spinal Accessory Mortor

The spinal accessory nerve is evaluated by testing the sternomastoid and trapezius muscles.   The sternomastoid muscles are tested by asking the patient to turn his head to one side or the other against resistance applied by the examiner.   The examiner should palpate these muscles as they are brought into play and compare the tone on the two sides. The left sternomastoid muscle turns the head to the right and vice versa.   The trapezius muscle is tested by asking the patient to shrug his shoulders.

CN XII   Examination of Tongue Movement

The hypoglossal nerve which is the motor nerve of the tongue is tested by asking the patient to protrude his tongue and to move it from side to side.   Unilateral injury results in paralysis, fasciculations and atrophy of the muscles of one half of the tongue. When the tongue is protruded it deviates towards the paralyzed side.   The patient should push out one cheek with his tongue and the tone of the tongue muscles may be palpated through the cheek.

THE MOTOR EXAMINATION

Motor functions to be tested include strength of individual muscles and muscle groups, coordination, gait and reflexes.

The examination should begin with careful observation of the patient.   His gait should be observed for unsteadiness or swaying, inequality of movement of either lower extremity, abnormal posture etc.   The arm swing should be equal bilaterally.   The patient is then asked to walk forward on his heels, toes, and in tandem fashion placing one foot directly in front of the other (see Fig. 3).   Awkwardness or inability to perform these various gaits may be caused by either underlying weakness or lack of coordination.   The patient is then seated and asked to extend his arms and legs in front of him and to close his eyes.   If weakness is present downward drift of an arm or leg may occur.   Upward drift of an extremity usually implies a loss of position sense of the extremity.   Next the upper extremity is evaluated beginning at the shoulder.   The patient is requested to elevate and lower his arm while the examiner applies resistance in the opposite direction.   The shoulder is also tested for forward and backward motion.   Flexion and extension, pronasion and supination of

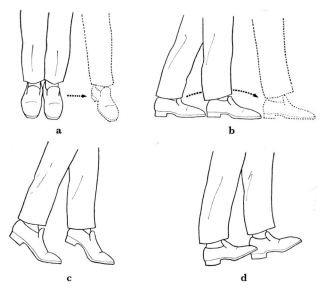

Fig. 3 Evaluation of gait.

a: Tandem walking. The patient is asked to side step.

b: Heel to toe. The paitent is asked to walk by placing the heel of one foot directly in front of the toe of the other foot and then to repeat this process.

c: Toe walking. The patient is asked to walk on his toes.

d: Heel walking. The patient is asked to walk on his heels.

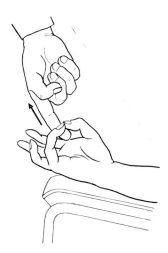

Fig. 4 The "circle" test.

The patient is asked to form a circle with his thumb and little finger. The examiner tries to pull this circle apart by exerting upward pressure with his index finger. The arrow indicates the direction of motion of the examiner's finger.

the arm are tested. At the wrist, flexion and extension are examined. Thumb abduction, adduction, palmar abduction etc. as well as flexion and extension of the thumb and finger should be tested. As shown in Fig. 4 palmar flexion of the thumb may be evaluated by instructing the patient to form a ring with his thumb and little finger. The examiner tries to "open" this ring using his index finger as shown. Handwriting is a good test of the fine motor control of the upper extremity. Hip, knee, ankle and foot extension, flexion, abduction and adduction are also examined.

1. Tests of Coordination and Balance

Rapid alternating movements: The patient is instructed to tap the fingers of one hand on the palm of the other, pat his knee alternately with the flexor and extensor surfaces of his hand and to tap his foot.   These movements are compared bilaterally.

Next he is instructed to alternately touch the examiner's finger and then his nose. (The examiner's finger is moved into various places in front of the patient during this test.) Next with his eyes closed the patient is instructed to touch his nose.   He is asked to touch his heel to his knee and run his heel down his shin.

The patient is also tested for past-pointing, which may occur in vestibular disorders. (refer to "the Past-pointing Test").

The patient is next asked to sit on the edge of a chair with his eyes closed and arms extended.   The examiner pushes against the patient in one direction or another to test his recovery from this push displacement.   ROMBERG's test is performed with the eyes open and closed.

2. Muscle Tone

The patient's limbs should be moved by the examiner while the muscles are palpated in order to evaluate muscle tone.   Tremor or fasciculations should be noted.

3. Deep Tendon Reflexes

Reflexes commonly tested are the jaw, biceps, triceps, radial, knee and ankle jerks. Reflexes should be fairly brisk and equal bilaterally.

4. The Babinski Reflex

The bottom of the foot should be lightly stroked from the back to the front.   A positive response occurs when the big toe elevates and the other toes flare.   Positive response is indicative of loss of upper motor neuron control.

Motor deficits may occur with lesions in the central nervous system, spinal roots or nerves or peripheral nerves.   In general, central dysfunction causes a pattern of weakness and consequent poor motor performance.   An example is the contralateral hemiplegia of unilateral cerebral or brainstem dysfunction.   There is no primary atrophy of the apparently weak muscles.   In contrast a lesion of a peripheral nerve or root will cause primary muscle weakness of the innervated muscle in question and atrophy and fasciculations will ensue.

THE SENSORY EXAMINATION

Modalities to be tested are touch, pain, temperature, vibration, and position sense. The body surface should be thoroughly evaluated bilaterally and the bilateral responses compared.   The value of double simultaneous stimulation in evaluating the sensory status cannot be overemphasized.   By applying equal stimuli to homonomous parts of the body subtle defects which may be overlooked during single stimulation may be revealed.

Dull versus sharp sensation is evaluated by alternately touching the patient with the examiner's finger and the sharp end of a safety-pin.   Pain is evaluated by using the sharp end of the pin and inquiring about the quality of the pain sensation produced (Fig. 5 a).   Pinprick sensation should be equal bilaterally.   As shown in Fig. 5 b, the position sense of the individual fingers as well as of the big toe is evaluated by moving the digit being examined up and down several times, stopping either in the elevated or depressed position and asking the patient if the digit is up or down.   If the position sense is intact in the peripheral digits it is almost certainly intact at more central joints.   If an abnormality is present, progressively more central joints should be tested i.e. first fingers, then wrist, elbow, in order to evaluate the severity of the dysfunction.

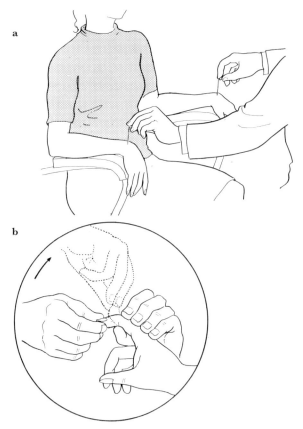

Fig. 5   The sensory examination.
a: Double simultaneous pain test.   The examiner lightly places the points of two pins on the
patient's forearms and asks the patient to compare the sensations.
b: Position sense.   The examiner fixes the second and third digits with one hand and manipu-
lates the first digit with his other hand.   The patient (with his eyes closed) is asked to report the
direction of motion i.e. up or down.   The arrow indicates the direction of motion.

Vibration sense is tested by applying a vibrating tuning fork to the patient's fingers and
bony prominences.

Temperature sense is tested by touching the subject with a metal object which should be
perceived as cool.

The value of a careful sensory examination lies in the evaluation of the pattern of sensory
deficit in combination with any motor defects and positive history.   Dissociation of sensation, i.e. loss of pain and temperature on one side of the body while touch and position
sense are spared, sensory levels, or unilateral sensory losses are all part of specific disease
complexes.

APPLICATION OF THE EXAMINATION

A few selected syndromes will be discussed.

Caution is to be urged in the interpretation of the following "syndromes" to be presented.
The occurrence of associated signs and symptoms in exactly the "classical textbook" form
is the exception rather than the rule.   The most reasonable course of diagnosis to be followed is to consider the signs and symptoms as well as the time course of the illness and

then to evaluate what area of the nervous system is involved.   Attempts to force the diagnosis along the lines of classic neurology are usually unsuccessful if the results of the examination and history are carefully considered.

1. Medulla Oblongata

The arterial circulation of the medulla has been divided into medial and lateral divisions. Disturbance of the blood flow by the occlusion of a branch of the vertebral or the posterior inferior cerebellar artery can produce softening or infarction of the lateral area of the medulla.   A prodrome of intermittent malaise and dizziness may be present, but the onset of severe symptoms is usually sudden and consists of any combination of the following; nausea, vomiting, vertigo, difficulty in swallowing and talking, and impaired coordination or balance on the side ipsilateral to the lesion with impaired sensation of pain and temperature on the side of the face ipsilateral to the lesion, and on the side of the body contralateral to the lesion.   An ipsilateral Horner's syndrome may be present.   Difficulty in swallowing and talking is due to damage to the nuclei or nerve fibers of the IXth or Xth nerve producing ipsilateral weakness of the palate, pharynx and vocal cord.   The vertigo and nausea may be due to the involvement of the vestibular nuclei while the impaired coordination is due to a lesion of the inferior cerebellar peduncle.   The loss of sensation in the face is secondary to the involvement of the descending root of the Vth nucleus while pain and temperature loss on the contralateral hemibody may be attributed to damage to lateral spinothalamic tract.   The medial lemniscus carrying the fibers for fine touch and proprioception is undamaged, therefore these functions are intact.   Recovery from damage to this area of the brain stem is usually gradual and incomplete.   In addition some patients may be left with a residual burning pain (hyperesthesia) in the areas of the original sensory loss.

Even though nausea, vomiting and vertigo may be the presenting symptoms of this illness the presence of sensory and motor losses should clearly delineate this complex from peripheral labyrinthine disease.

2. Cerebellopontine Angle

Acoustic neurinoma (cerebello-pontine angle tumor):   Tumors of the VIIIth nerve lying within the internal auditory canal usually produce a sense of imbalance and a hearing loss secondary to compression of the VIIIth nerve.   These symptoms may or may not be noticed by the patient and these tumors often grow to a large size before any dysfunction becomes apparent.   With the growth of the tumor there are symptoms and signs of involvement of the nearby cranial nerves, and of the brain stem secondary to damage by compression.   If the patient does not seek medical attention when the tumor is small, he may often present later with vague complaints of dizziness, unsteady gait or falling.   On examination the labyrinth on the affected side is usually unresponsive to caloric stimulation. The ipsilateral corneal reflex is commonly lost and there may be other sensory losses in the area of distribution of the Vth nerve.   Involvement of the facial nerve is sometimes noted as weakness of the facial muscles.   This weakness may become apparent upon vigorous testing and comparison of the strength of the facial muscles bilaterally.   If the tumor is very large the brain stem may be compressed and pushed to the opposite side.   Once again the presence of motor and sensory involvement should indicate the location of the pathology.

3. Pons

Interruption of the blood supply or the presence of a primary or metastatic tumor may give rise to a dysfunction of the pons.   Signs and symptoms of pontine damage include paralysis of the VIth and VIIth nerves giving rise to an ipsilateral loss of eye abduction and perhaps ipsilateral conjugate gaze paralysis and loss of ipsilateral facial movement. Loss of pontocerebellar fibers may cause ataxia and pyramidal tracts cause hemi- or quadriparesis. A lesion of the medial lemniscus will cause sensory disturbances. In addition consciousness may be variably impaired. Pontine syndromes should be individually evaluated as to the site or sites of the lesion as classification into categories is difficult.

4. Midbrain

Dysfunction of the pretectal area of the midbrain may be caused by tumors of the pineal gland, third ventricle, or sylvian aqueduct. If the aqueduct is stenotic eventual dysfunction of the pretectal area may result and further, if acute blockage of the aqueduct occurs, consciousness will usually be impaired. Eye signs associated with dysfunction of the area of the pretectum-posterior commissure include a disturbance of vertical gaze (upward gaze is usually more severely affected than downward gaze), pupillary abnormalities, paresis of convergence and, rarely, the retraction type of nystagmus. These signs including loss of consciousness may sometimes be reversed if prompt treatment is undertaken.

Examination of Hearing or Audiometry

The examination of hearing is an integral part of the neuro-otological examination and is important for the following reasons.

(1) The acoustic end organ (the cochlea) and the equilibrium end organ (the otolithic organs and semicircular canals) are situated close to each other in the labyrinth. Pathological processes in the labyrinth therefore frequently affect both of these sets of organs together.

(2) On the contrary, in the brainstem the central pathways for the acoustic and the vestibular systems are separated. Central lesions, accordingly, usually do not affect both functions equally, therefore isolated dysfunction of one of these two may indicate a central lesion.

(3) Also a lesion in one or the other of these two systems may sometimes provoke symptoms or signs definitely indicating the site of the lesion. This may be useful for local diagnosis in the other system.

Neuro-otology covers the areas connected with the eighth cranial nerve, i.e. both the acoustic and the vestibular systems. In neurological diagnosis, however, the vestibular system has traditionally contributed more to diagnosis than has the acoustic system. This is still so at the present, in spite of the recent remarkable developments in audiology.

Some of these recent advances in audiology may be listed as follows: (1) definite diagnosis of conductive deafness, (2) positive indication of deafness due to a hair cell lesion in the inner ear, (3) correlation of hearing threshold curves with the causes of deafness, (4) Indication of retrolabyrinthine deafness by over-threshold hearing tests.

The technical descriptions and rather sophisticated methods used in audiological examinations are omitted from this book, but several diagnostically important methods and results of examination will be briefly described:

1. Measurement of pure tone threshold
2. Examination of the recruitment phenomenon
3. Speech discrimination or articulation tests
4. Monaural speech integration tests
5. Binaural speech integration tests

MEASUREMENT OF PURE TONE THRESHOLD

This is the basic and most important audiometry test. The pure tone thresholds are determined by both the air and bone conduction methods. The threshold of air and bone conduction is routinely examined with an audiometer. The threshold curves of air conduction have typical shapes some of which are classically related to different causes of deafness, such as deafness from acoustic or head trauma, aging, streptomycin intoxication, etc. (Fig. 6). The threshold difference between air and bone conductions is called the air-bone gap, or A-B gap and this gap indicates sound conductive versus sound perceptive deafness. The deafness from acoustic neurinoma, for example, is sound perceptive but not conductive.

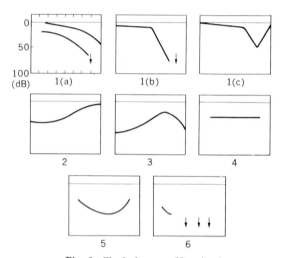

Fig. 6 Typical types of hearing loss.
1(a): Gradual high tone loss: streptomycin ototoxicity, presbycusis, etc., 1(b): Abrupt high tone loss, 1(c): C_5-dip: acoustic trauma, etc., 2: Low tone loss, 3: High and low tone loss; 2 and 3: Ménière's disease, 4: Flat loss, 5: Middle tone loss, 6: Complete deafness.

The Weber test is performed by applying the bone conduction vibrator at the midline of the skull. In patients with unilateral hearing loss the sound delivered through this vibrator may be perceived louder in one or the other ear. The sound is usually louder in the conductive deaf ear, and softer in the perceptive deaf ear.

EXAMINATION OF THE RECRUITMENT PHENOMENON

The recruitment phenomenon is believed to be a phenomenon caused by diseased hair cells in the inner ear. To detect the phenomenon, two important test methods are used:

1. Alternating Binaural Loudness Balance Test (ABLB Test, Fowler, 1936)

When the threshold of hearing on one side is significantly elevated (more than 20 dB) compared to that on the other side, this test is applicable. When the thresholds of hearing of both sides are different by a certain dB level the loudness balance is always obtained with this amount of dB difference in conductive deafness, i.e. when the threshold difference at 1000 Hz is 40 dB, then the perceived loudness of the 80 dB sound on the deaf ear will be balanced with that of a 40 dB sound on the side of the healthy ear.

In a certain type of inner ear deafness, however, loudness balance will be achieved with a 90 dB sound for either side in spite of the threshold difference of 40 dB, for example (Fig. 7). This is a frequent finding in Ménière's disease and is called a positive recruitment phenomenon. This is attributed by many investigators to diseased hair cells of the organ of Corti. Sometimes, however, balancing the loudness on both sides is not easy for the test subject, especially when the tones heard on the diseased ear appear distorted, turbid, or muffled.

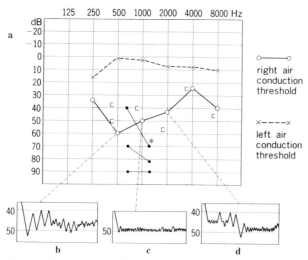

Fig. 7 Audiometric findings in a case of Ménière's disease.
Female, age 45. A typical third stage Ménière's disease (see Fig. 9). Air conduction loss can be seen on the right side. Bone conduction thresholds are also elevated. The ABLB test indicates recruitment at 1000 Hz(※) and the Békésy audiometry shows a diminished amplitude at 1000 and 2000Hz, and the maximum speech discrimination is 58%. a: pure tone audiometry results; b,c,d: Békésy audiograms at 500, 1000 and 2000Hz respectively.

2. Békésy Audiometry (BÉKÉSY, 1947)

Pure tone threshold curves are automatically recorded with the Békésy audiometer. The narrow tracking in the Békésy audiogram is believed to be a phenomenon similar to the recruitment detected by ABLB test.

The threshold measured by applying interrupted tones through the Békésy audiometer is different from that measured by continuous tones in some specific conditions. JERGER (1960–1) classified the findings into five types: Type 1 where the thresholds measured by interrupted and continuous tones are the same; Type 2 where the threshold measured by interrupted tones is lower by 5–20 dB than the threshold with continuous tones in the middle and the high tone areas; Type 3 where the threshold measured by continuous tones shifts by 40–50 dB within 60 seconds, while the threshold with interrupted tones stays constant; Type 4 where the threshold with interrupted tones is lower than that with continuous tones even in low tone areas; and Type 5 where the continuous tone threshold is lower than the interrupted tone threshold. Type 1 may indicate normal or conductive deafness, Type 2, 3, and 4 indicate inner ear or VIIth nerve deafness and Type 5, nonorganic deafness.

Fatigue in hearing is conveniently tested by utilizing a Békésy type audiometer. It is called the Temporary Threshold Shift (TTS) and is positive in cases with retrolabyrinthine, especially VIIIth nerve lesions.

Ménière's disease is believed to be due to a lesion in the labyrinth and it is important

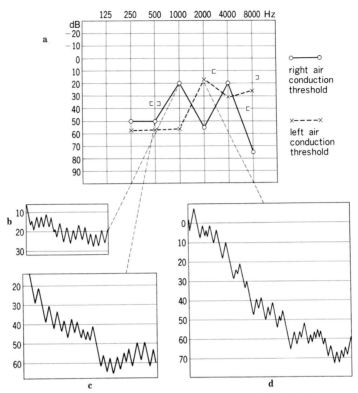

Fig. 8 Audiometric findings in a case of retrolabyrinthine deafness.
Male, age 34.   The unusual air conduction threshold curves may indicate a difficult threshold measurement in this case.   Békésy audiograms (b–d) show threshold shifts especially in c (500Hz in the right ear) and d(2000Hz in the left ear).   Maximum speech discrimination is 6% at 80dBSL on the right and 14% at 90dBSL on the left.

to demonstrate labyrinthine deafness in order to confirm the diagnosis of this disease. Pure tone threshold curves in a typical Ménière's disease are shown in the Fig. 7.   The ABLB test shows a positive recruitment and automatic audiometry with continuous tones shows a diminished amplitude.   The degree of deafness in Ménière's disease usually varies with the attacks of vertigo, and is manifested mostly in the low tone areas.   During the attacks, the threshold is high and between attacks it is low.   When vertiginous episodes occur repeatedly, the threshold is usually elevated by degrees and finally reaches a high degree of deafness (Fig. 9).

SPEECH DISCRIMINATION OR ARTICULATION TESTS

The speech discrimination test is important both for detecting the social adaptability of a subject and for diagnostic purposes as well.   Usually conductive deafness does not affect speech discrimination.   Perceptive deafness due to inner ear lesions has a moderate effect on speech discrimination but the deafness due to lesions in the central nervous system may most significantly affect the speech discrimination score.

MONAURAL SPEECH INTEGRATION TESTS

There are at present two kinds of distorted words available for testing, 1) filtered sounds

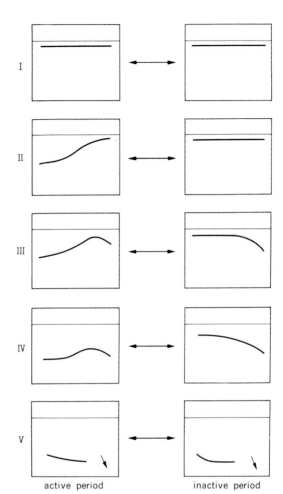

active period   inactive period

Fig. 9 Five disease stages of Ménière's disease.

Hearing impairment in Ménière's disease increases during repeated vertiginous attacks and finally approaches complete deafness. Typical Ménière's disease is characterized by a low tone deafness as seen in II of the left column. The low tone deafness during or after an attack may return to normal as seen in II on the right. When the attacks are repeated, thresholds are gradually elevated as illustrated from I to V. Thus, Ménière's disease may be divided into five stages (I–V) which can be specified by air conduction audiometry. At each stage during attacks the low tone deafness is more pronounced (active period), while between attacks it is less pronounced (inactive period). Treatment of Ménière's disease should be started during the earlier stages of the disease.

2) interrupted sounds. The discrimination of the two is believed to be useful for the differentiation of labyrinthine and retrolabyrinthine deafness.

BINAURAL HEARING TESTS

There are three kinds of binaural hearing tests clinically available: 1) directional hearing tests, 2) binaural speech integration tests, 3) binaural discrimination. All of these often give positive results in retro-labyrinthine deafness. The diagnostic significance of these tests are still to be developed.

Equilibrium Function Tests

LIMB AND TRUNK SIGNS OF DISEQUILIBRIUM

The labyrinth exerts a strong tonic influence on the motor system including the eye, trunk, and limb muscles and helps maintain the equilibrium of the body. If one labyrinth becomes abnormal, the balance between the left and right labyrinths may be impaired and cause disequilibrium of the body. When such a patient is asked to stand with his eyes closed and his arms extended forward, he may assume a characteristic posture called the "discus-thrower position".

For example, if the left labyrinth is severely damaged, the signs may be listed as follows (Fig. 10).

1. Eye deviation (slow phase) to the left, resulting in spontaneous nystagmus (quick phase) to the right.
2. Head turning to the left.
3. Trunk twisting to the left.
4. Deviation of both arms to the left accompanied by a raising of the right arm and a lowering of the left arm.
5. Falling tendency to the left.
6. Deviation of gait to the left.

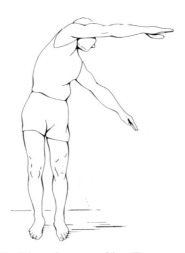

Fig. 10 Discus-thrower position (FRENZEL, 1955).

It can be said that one purpose of equilibrium function tests is to look for the above-mentioned eye, trunk, and limbs signs and evaluate their severity. If bilateral labyrinthine damage to an almost equal extent is present, the dysfunction may appear as a disturbance of the righting reflex, i.e. an unsteadiness of the body in all directions.

Cerebellar lesions can also cause severe equilibrium disturbance including impaired ability to stand or walk even with the eyes open in light. This disability is often accompanied by ataxia of the limbs (i.e. errors in rate, range, direction and force of voluntary movements).

Effects of unilateral labyrinthine lesions are usually manifested bilaterally; however, an unilateral cerebellar lesion will often produce only ipsilateral signs.

EXAMINATION

1. The Standing Test

The standing test is performed in the following sequence of increasing difficulty.   The patient is asked to stand with both feet close together with the eyes open and then closed. Subsequently he is asked to stand alternatively on one leg and on the other with the eyes open and then closed.

The examiner should observe any swaying of the body or falling tendency.   In labyrinthine, vestibular nerve, and presumably vestibular nuclei lesions there is coincidence of the direction of falling tendency with that of the slow phase of spontaneous nystagmus.   When the patient is asked to turn his head to the right or left, the falling tendency in cases with labyrinthine ataxia may change in accordance with the direction of slow phase of the spontaneous nystagmus.   Whether this occurs as a result of a labyrinthine lesion is questionable.   A patient with acute unilateral loss of labyrinthine function may partially recover in a few months and be able to stand on one foot with the eyes open, but be unable to stand on one foot with the eyes closed.   If a patient is able to stand on each leg with his eyes closed, he may be regarded as essentially normal and other vestibular function tests are not necessary.   In this sense, standing on one leg can be regarded as a screening test for disequilibrium.

Several procedures have been suggested to increase the sensitivity of the standing test, such as standing with one foot in front of the other (Mann, 1912) or by using the Jendrassik maneuver for distracting the patient's attention.   However, the above mentioned standing test alone is sufficient to detect disequilibrium.

2. The Walking (or Gait) Test

The patient is asked to walk straight forward or backward with his eyes blindfolded. Staggering or deviation of gait from the straight forward direction should be noted.

3. The Stepping Test

The test is carried as follows, after Fukuda (1959).   The patient is securely blindfolded and is asked to stand in the center of three concentric circles with diameters of 0.5, 1.0 and 1.5 meters respectively.   He is then asked to extend his arms forward and to march in place.   (It may be preferable to have the patient remove his shoes.)   The total number of steps, 50 or 100, are performed at normal walking speed.   During stepping the examiner should observe for swaying of the body, change of the head position relative to the body and deviation of the arms in the horizontal or vertical plane.   The final position after completion of stepping and path followed from the starting position are recorded on a chart (Fig. 11).   The angle of body rotation around the vertical axis ("d" in Fig. 11) is also measured.

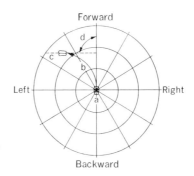

Fig. 11   Record of the result of the stepping test.
a: The starting position;   b: The path followed from a to c;   c: The final position;   d: The angle of body rotation

Body rotation of more than 30 degrees, backward displacement of the final position or forward displacement of more than 1 meter are regarded as abnormal. As mentioned, the direction of body rotation may coincide with that of the slow phase of labyrinthine nystagmus if present.

4. Goniometer Test

The horizontal board of the goniometer is gradually inclined forward, backward, right and left, and the angle, at which the patient is unable to maintain his footing on the board, is measured. This test is performed first with the eyes open and next with the eyes closed.

It has been said that there is a wide individual variation on normal subjects, which makes the test results difficult to interpret. The following criteria for abnormality were suggested by FUKUDA and HINOKI (1965); the angle, at which the footing is lost, is 15 degrees or less in either of the four directions; the difference between the angle with the open and closed eyes is 5 degrees or more; the difference between the angle of inclination to the right and the left side is 5 degrees or more.

HONJO and FURUKAWA (1957) devised an electrically driven goniometer in order to increase the reliability of the test results.

5. The Past-pointing Test

The patient is seated in a chair and places one hand palm down on his knee with the index finger stretched out. He is asked to raise his arm and touch the examiner's finger held in front of the patient at a level of his shoulder. The test is performed first with the eyes open and next with the eyes closed. Deviation of the patient's finger from the examiner's to either side is observed.

Past-pointing in a labyrinthine lesion will be manifested by both arms, while in a cerebellar lesion it may be present on the affected side only.

6. Vertical Writing with Eyes Closed or the Blindfolded Vertical Writing Test (FUKUDA, 1959)

The patient is asked to sit on a chair facing a desk with his body upright and to place his left hand on his knee. Using a pencil with a soft lead or a felt tipped pen held with the right hand (or the left hand for a left-handed subject) 4 or 5 Chinese letters or capital alphabetical letters such as ABCDE are written vertically on graph paper. (The arm should be fully extended in front of the subject and the arm and body should not touch the desk.) Each letter should be as large as 3×3 or 5×5 cm.

This test is first conducted with the eyes open and next in a similar way with the eyes securely blindfolded. In the latter case the test should be repeated more than two times in order to ascertain whether the finding is reproducible. The greatest deviation of written letters is measured in degrees from a line drawn vertically from the middle of the top letter. If a deviation of more than 10 degrees is found solely in the letters written during the blindfolded test, unilateral labyrinthine lesion may be indicated (Fig. 12 a). On the other hand, a patient with cerebellar ataxia may write unrecognizable letters instead of letters showing a definite slant (Fig. 12b). If a unilateral cerebellar lesion is present, the percentage of abnormality is different depending on the affected side (i.e. a right-handed subject with a left cerebellar hemisphere lesion may perform this test rather normally).

The positive rate in patients with acoustic neurinoma was 58% (7 out of 12 cases) with a left sided tumor and 89% (8 out of 9 cases) with a right sided tumor, when the tests were conducted only with the right hand (UEMURA et al., 1963). This indicates that the test must be conducted with both hands. In this regard it is pointed out that SAYK (1964) introduced the synergy-writing test as a cerebellar function test, in which a number 3 is drawn with the right and left hands alternately.

The above-mentioned tests with the exception of the goniometer test have an advantage for clinical practice in that special equipment is not necessary. Careful attention should

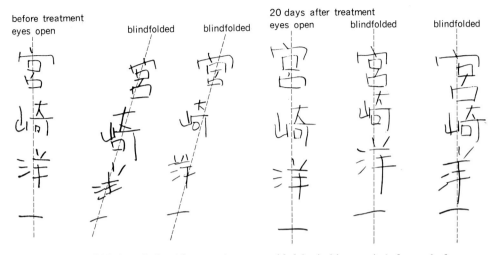

Fig. 12 a The blindfolded vertical writing tests in a case with labyrinthine ataxia before and after treatment

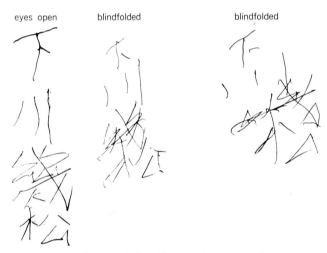

Fig. 12 b The blindfolded vertical writing tests in a case with cerebellar ataxia.

be paid to the testing procedure and its interpretation, since the results are apt to be disturbed by accidental or volitional testing errors.   To prevent these errors, the results obtained must be consistently reproducible when the tests are repeated.   Even if it is assumed that the results indicate some imbalance of the vestibulospinal reflex, the relation between the side of labyrinthine pathology and the direction of the body deviation is not so simple as that between the side of the lesion and the direction of nystagmus.   This complex might be ascribed to the existence of hypercompensation following the process of compensation (WODAK and FISCHER, 1924) or the emergence of a tonic deviation directed oppositely between the "stages of coordination and of disturbance" (FUKUDA, 1959b).

In conclusion, examination for limb and trunk signs are necessary for revealing the character and severity of disequilibrium, but they are limited at present to the purpose of deciding the side and location of the pathology.

SIGNS RELATED TO ABNORMAL EYE MOVEMENTS

EXAMINATION OF SPONTANEOUS AND EVOKED NYSTAGMUS

If some central nervous or vestibular dysfunction is associated with a disturbance of the perception of the spatial orientation of the body, this subjective manifestation of the dysfunction is vertigo. If "true vertigo" is present, spontaneous nystagmus should be present as an objective manifestation of this dysfunction: In fact in patients with "true vertigo", spontaneous nystagmus is usually present. Spontaneous nystagmus is not under voluntary control, i.e. it can not be willfully modified by the patient. This is a fundamental difference between the findings from the examination of the eyes and those of the body. For example, limb tremors can often be partially controlled by patients, and deviation or staggering elicited during the stepping test can be artificially modified.

The diagnostic importance of spontaneous nystagmus is that it may be possible to localize the lesion or area of dysfunction responsible for the nystagmus. There is an extremely large variety of different types of spontaneous nystagmus but close observation can classify these types according to the direction, plane of beat, amplitude, frequency, response to different head positions, and so on.

There are three different possible sign and symptom combinations, namely, 1) only vertigo is present, 2) only spontaneous nystagmus is present, and 3) both vertigo and spontaneous nystagmus are present. When spontaneous nystagmus and vertigo exist, the classification of this nystagmus can be correlated with the vertigo, and integrated into a final diagnosis. For example, labyrinthine lesions of acute onset are usually accompanied by both vertigo and spontaneous nystagmus. Spontaneous nystagmus can be only horizontal, rotatory, or horizontal-rotatory. The characteristics of spontaneous nystagmus indicate a group of diseases, while a disease indicates the possible range of types of spontaneous nystagmus.

1. The Classification of Spontaneous Nystagmus

A description of nystagmus is necessary for classification purposes. The following are the basic terms important in clinical descriptions of nystagmus.

(a) Beat mode: jerking, pendular, irregular.

(b) Association of the movements of both eyes: associated or dissociated.

(c) Plane of movement: horizontal, rotating, vertical, horizontal-rotating, vertical-rotating, diagonal.

(d) Direction (the direction of the quick phase of jerking nystagmus): right, left, upward, downward, clockwise, counterclockwise.

(e) Amplitude and frequency: large, medium or small amplitude; high, medium or low frequency.

(f) Duration: long or short lasting; transient.

(g) Changes: declining, augmenting; rhythmical, arrhythmical.

(h) Influences of head position or head position change: positional or positioning nystagmus.

(i) Rare conditions: seesaw nystagmus, periodically alternating nystagmus, convergence nystagmus, divergence nystagmus, latent or unimacular nystagmus, retraction nystagmus.

(j) External stimuli alter spontaneous nystagmus or induce nystagmus: optic, optokinetic; vestibular, labyrinthine (galvanic, caloric, rotatory: per-rotatory and post-rotatory); fistular.

There are many different systems for classifying spontaneous nystagmus in the literature. The following classification (SUZUKI, 1971) is however convenient for clinical purposes:

1) Physiological nystagmus
   Pathologic physiological nystagmus
   Pathological nystagmus

Physiological nystagmus is that nystagmus which appears in normal subjects, for example during head motion. It may be present to an abnormal degree and therefore is considered pathologic physiological nystagmus. Pathological nystagmus is nystagmus not seen in normal subjects under any conditions, and is thus different from pathologic physiological nystagmus.

2) Spontaneous nystagmus
   Positional nystagmus   Positioning nystagmus
   Evoked nystagmus (experimentally induced nystagmus)

Spontaneous, positional and positioning nystagmus are "pathological nystagmus". Experimentally induced nystagmus is "physiological nystagmus" and refers to nystagmus induced by rotatory, caloric, optokinetic or some other stimulation.

3) Vestibular nystagmus
   Non-vestibular nystagmus
   Ophthalmogenic nystagmus

Nystagmus from the vestibular system, central and peripheral, may be called vestibular nystagmus to distinguish it from non-vestibular nystagmus. Nystagmus from lesions in the visual and oculomotor systems is non-vestibular nystagmus, and includes all so-called congenital, idiopathic and related nystagmus, i.e. ophthalmogenic nystagmus.

4) Nystagmus during gaze (gaze nystagmus)

Nystagmus is present without visual input, for example, during darkness or with the eyes closed. This type of nystagmus may be called non-gaze nystagmus.

Usually non-vestibular nystagmus is a type of gaze nystagmus, while vestibular nystagmus is a type of nystagmus present with or without vision. Gaze nystagmus and nystagmus in the absence of vision may be differentiated clinically as well as theoretically.

5) Jerking nystagmus
   Pendular nystagmus

Jerking nystagmus has two phases, the slow and the quick phases while the phases of typical pendular nystagmus are of equal amplitude and velocity; thus the name pendular is applied.

6) Horizontal nystagmus   Horizontal-rotating nystagmus,
   Vertical nystagmus   Vertical-rotating nystagmus,
   Rotating nystagmus   Diagonal nystagmus

The identification of the beating plane of any nystagmus is important in localizing causative lesions.

7) Nystagmus of low frequency and large amplitude
   Nystagmus of high frequency and small amplitude

Low frequency large amplitude nystagmus is usually due to central lesions while the high frequency small amplitude nystagmus is usually due to labyrinthine lesions. Nystagmus due to central lesions can, however, occasionally be of the latter type.

2. Method of Examination
a. Gaze and fixation nystagmus

Method. The subject is asked to look at a point more than 50 cm distant.   The directions of gaze to be tested are forward, lateral to the right and to the left, upward and downward (Fig. 13).*   The degree of lateral gaze should be about 30 degrees from the midline.   Extreme lateral gaze of more than 30 degrees could induce physiological end-position nystagmus.   The test is conducted with both eyes open, and then with each eye alternately covered.   If nystagmus appears when one eye is covered, it is called latent or unimacular nystagmus.   This is mostly congenital and of central origin.   Although the standard testing distance between the eyes and the point of fixation is usually about 50 cm, fixation at a very close point and also at a very far point may induce nystagmus or have some influence on nystagmus.   This should be noted.

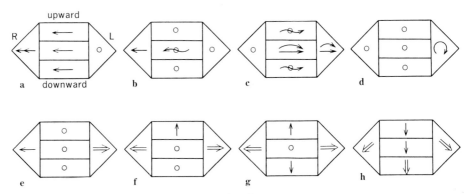

Fig. 13 Examples of gaze nystagmus.
Examples shown in the hexagonal diagrams (a–d) generally result from peripheral vestibular lesions and may be called peripheral or P type.   Examples in the diagrams (e–h) result from cases of central lesions and may be called central or C type.

When one gazes at a near point, the eyes converge.   Convergence and upward gaze frequently are slightly weak in old people.   These abnormalities may be regarded as an impairment within the physiological range in patients over 60 years of age.   Pathological impairment of convergence or upward gaze is believed due to lesions in the tectum or the pretectal area.**

Diagnostic significance

(1)   Gaze nystagmus is an important pathological finding and it should be carefully documented.   If the nystagmus is very fine and the examiner is uncertain of its classification, this should also be noted as such by writing down the sign ⌒ or ⌒ on the diagram indicating the uncertainess of the finding.   Although this nystagmus may have no direct diagnostic significance it may be an important ancillary finding.

---

  * Before secondary for nystagmus, eye movements themselves have to be carefully examined: 1) conjugate motion of the two eyes, 2) limitation of lateral, up and down gaze, and 3) convergence are examined. Observation of each eye should be carefully performed both singly and during conjugate gaze.

 ** Gazing is an important function of the oculomotor system especially for animals with binocular vision, i.e. man and monkey.   During gaze, the eyes must converge for stereoscopic vision.   The eye movements required for binocular fixation and gaze must necessarily be performed very precisely and are accordingly very well controlled by CNS mechanisms.   The nystagmus which is believed to be due to dysfunction of the gaze mechanism is also called gaze-paretic nystagmus.   A good example is the infrequent and large amplitude nystagmus directed to the side of the lesion in the case of a pontine angle tumor.

(2) Gaze nystagmus may be divided into: 1) that in a unilateral horizontal direction, 2) that in a bilateral horizontal direction and 3) that in directions other than horizontal. Among these, unilateral gaze nystagmus is the most common and can be both of labyrinthine and central origin. Bilateral gaze nystagmus is not uncommon and is believed to be of central origin. This bilateral gaze nystagmus can be symmetric or asymmetric. Gaze nystagmus in non-horizontal directions is less common and is believed to be also of central origin.

Bilateral gaze nystagmus of a small amplitude and/or short duration is usually non-pathologic and may appear in normal subjects especially if they are physically weak or exhausted. It may also appear when the subject maintains lateral gaze for a long period of time, or holds an extreme lateral gaze. It is very common after barbiturate ingestion.

There may also be transient nystagmic eye movements when the visual target is moved too quickly, or immediately after the eyes fixate a target. These cannot be regarded as pathological if they appear as isolated findings.*

Cases with pontine angle tumors often have bilateral gaze nystagmus of an asymmetric nature; large and infrequent to the side of the tumor, and small and frequent to the other side. This is called "Bruns' nystagmus"(Fig. 125).

Basilar impression is a congenital malformation in the area around the foramen magnum which may not become clinically apparent until adulthood. The symptoms of gait disturbance or imbalance may resemble cerebellar degenerative diseases. The condition usually shows marked downward beating vertical nystagmus as shown in Fig. 13-h. The degree of the malformation varies from case to case. Cases with less severe lesions show less intense vertical nystagmus which may be visible only behind Frenzel glasses or only after vertical positioning of the head from the sitting to the head-hanging position. Arnold Chiari malformation frequently has similar signs.

Congenital idiopathic nystagmus is a particular condition in which a remarkable nystagmus is frequently the only positive finding. Spontaneous nystagmus in these cases may be jerking or pendular in type, and is usually very active when the eyes are open in the light and is depressed when the eyes are covered or especially when they are closed.**

b. Nystagmus present without visual fixation, spontaneous nystagmus

In complete darkness, and/or with the eyes closed, there can be no visual fixation (therefore "seeing" or vision is interdicted). With no active images on the retina during these conditions, holding a steady visual line is difficult for the subject; this is believed to be due to the lack of visual feedback from the retina.

Even in normal subjects there may be slight tonic imbalance in the CNS between right and left or between up and down gaze directions. This tonic imbalance can be greater in pathological cases and, if present, may cause the eyes to deviate in darkness and slow

---

* Gaze nystagmus due to lateral gaze to the extreme lateral direction is called end-position nystagmus and may be regarded as physiological nystagmus. This end-position nystagmus shows great individual variation and is sensitive to the physical condition of the subject. A distinct nystagmus which appears with a lateral gaze of 30° or less from the midline is empirically believed to be pathological. The distinction between physiological and pathological gaze nystagmus is however arbitary, sometimes difficult and may be impossible. Whenever difficulty in identifying the findings becomes apparent, recording of the findings should be accompanied by comments or notes. Only discrete nystagmus with a sufficiently large amplitude which is easily identified can be said to be unequivocally pathological.

** The condition is believed to be due to a lesion in the oculomotor system. Accordingly, gaze function, optokinetic eye responses and other eye movements may be disturbed. These nystagmus waves as recorded by ENG have a characteristic appearance which is different from other kinds of jerking nystagmus.

If congenital nystagmus is present, a small intravenously applied dose of barbiturate may result in a remarkable cessation of the nystagmus and a concomitant improvement in visual acuity in the patient.

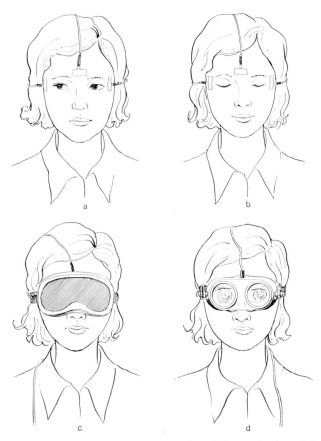

Fig. 14 Observation of nystagmus in the four different visual conditions.
a: The eyes open, gazing to the right; b: The eyes closed; c: The eyes open and covered;
d: The eyes open behind Frenzel glasses.
Electrodes attached for recording eye movements in the horizontal plane through an electrony-stagmograph.

tonic deviation will be corrected by a quick return movement to the original position. This slow and quick motion of the eyes may be repeated and become a jerking type of nystagmus.

Method. Clinically non-gaze nystagmus present without visual fixation is examined behind Frenzel glasses, however, electronystagmography is especially useful for recording this type of nystagmus, since recording is possible in complete darkness or with the eyes closed. Nystagmus in these condition may not be visually observed. Changes in alertness brought about by ordering the test subject to perform a calculation are valuable in eliciting very weak nystagmus.

A convenient analogy may be drawn between eye movements and a laboratory scale or balance. With the eyes open and spontaneous gaze occurring, the "balance" is in the "up" or disengaged position; when the eyes are closed or covered or vision is interrupted by Frenzel glasses, the balance is engaged and is extremely sensitive to unequal "weights" on one side or the other. These "weights" or inequalities in vestibular or central input to the oculomotor system, even though small, manifest themselves by nystagmic eye movements when vision is interdicted and the "balance is engaged".

Diagnostic significance. Spontaneous nystagmus is regarded as one of the important objective findings in vertigo, and is by itself a pathological finding.

Those cases with lesions in the labyrinth usually have spontaneous nystagmus of a non-gaze character. Ménière's disease, labyrinthitis of various nature, paroxysmal inner ear dysfunction and so on are included. When the imbalance is large, the nystagmus can be seen under gaze condition but it is much more intensive during "non-gaze" (Fig. 15). Spontaneous nystagmus is usually directed to the side of the lesion in the acute stage but in the chronic stage it is usually directed to the side contralateral to the lesion.

Cases with lesions in the CNS which generate the condition of tonic imbalance may also show spontaneous nystagmus of a non-gaze character. Directional preponderance of induced nystagmus is a condition which may generate spontaneous nystagmus as evoked by nystagmus tests during "non-gaze".

Directional preponderance (DP) of nystagmus is believed to be a condition which progresses to spontaneous nystagmus of a non-gaze character, i.e. weak non-gaze spontaneous nystagmus. The DP is revealed by several different kinds of examination, such as the subliminal rotation test, microcalorimetry, optokinetic after-nystagmus test, etc. There are, however, different opinions about whether DP of nystagmus is pathological when the condition is detected by a very sensitive examination method. Empirically, this author is of the opinion that spontaneous nystagmus revealed by relatively simple loading, such as applying mental calculation or changing head positions, is pathological. The DP detected by sensitive methods may not be pathological in and of itself. This may be called "physiological DP" in contrast to "pathological DP". The difference may be only a question of degree of the DP.

ENG recordings must be carefully examined, since spontaneous nystagmus is sometimes difficult to distinguish from eye blink artifact (see p. 55). This isespecially true of vertical recordings where the electrical record of the blinking is large. A definite conclusion about doubtful spontaneous nystagmus can be drawn from vertical ENG recordings only by adding other supporting data.

c. Positional nystagmus

When the subject assumes different head positions, vertigo may be augmented and nystagmus may be induced. This may occur in patients with no spontaneous vertigo complaints. The nystagmus which is induced in different head positions is called positional nystagmus, and is an important clinical finding in cases of vertigo or loss of balance.

Method. Examination of positional nystagmus is always performed during non-gaze, i.e. with Frenzel glasses.* Of the many different possible head positions, eleven are routinely tested. These include six head positions which are assumed while lying supine (Fig. 16 c) and five head positions which are assumed while sitting (Fig. 16 a). The latter positions are omitted in screening tests because of the lesser incidence of positional nystagmus in them. Positions with the head twisted to the right and left while sitting are also tested to examine the influence of neck twist apart from otolithic influences (Fig. 16 b).

The head position change should be performed as slowly as possible to avoid positioning or dynamic influences, and nystagmus in a particular head position should be observed for as long as 30 seconds or more when needed. When nystagmus is noticed, the nature of nystagmus such as the latency, the direction, the direction change of the nystagmus, etc. should be noted. The influence of repeating the same head position on the nystagmus evoked should also be noted; care is needed, as a positional nystagmus with a long latency and infrequent beats may be easily overlooked.

---

* The positional nystagmus test is performed under non-gaze because its purpose is to find any central imbalance reflected by the eye-position, "physiological balance", and not to evaluate the status of the oculomotor system. This "physiological balance" should be kept maximally sensitive by keeping the eyes open in darkness and focused at infinity.

amplitude
calibration: 10°

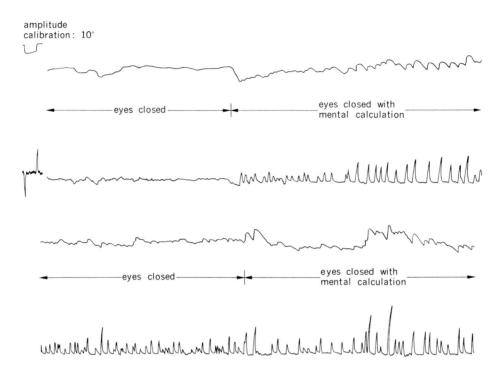

Fig. 15 ENG recordings of spontaneous nystagmus in a case of Ménière's disease affecting the right ear. No spontaneous nystagmus is seen with the eyes closed, however nystagmus was induced by mental calculation. Nystagmus is also present with the eyes open and covered both with and without mental calculation.

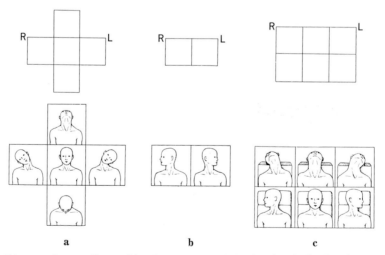

Fig. 16 Diagrams for recording positional nystagmus and the drawings indicating the corresponding head positions.
a: Positional nystagmus examination with the sitting position. The five different head positions with the body sitting are the head upright, the right-side down, the left-side-down, supine and prone.
b: Head-twisting to the right and the left with the body sitting. This procedure is for examining the effects of neck-twist on eye movements.
c: Positional nystagmus examination in the lying position. The six different head positions with the body supine are the head supine, the right-side-down, the left-side-down, the head-hanging, the head-hanging with the head twisted to the right and to the left.

Diagnostic Significance

(1) 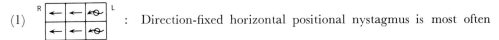 : Direction-fixed horizontal positional nystagmus is most often

encountered.   This indicates the existence of a lateralized condition, i.e. a lesion in the labyrinth or a lateralized lesion in the CNS.

(2) 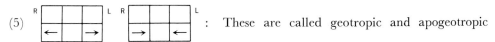 : Direction-fixed horizontal-rotating positional nystagmus which

may change its intensity in different head positions is frequently encountered in labyrinthine lesions.

(3) ⏐↓⏐ : Vertical-rotating positional nystagmus is seen relatively frequently.   This

may be caused by labyrinthine or central lesions.

When this type of nystagmus is small in amplitude, it may be noted either as pure vertical nystagmus or as pure rotating nystagmus, or as oblique nystagmus, any of which has implications different from that of the vertical-rotating type of nystagmus.

(4) ⏐⇓⏐ : Pure vertical positional nystagmus is always of central origin.   Since pure

vertical nystagmus is believed to be exclusively of central origin, it should be carefully identified.   Practically, only a large amplitude nystagmus can be noted as pure vertical nystagmus.

(5) 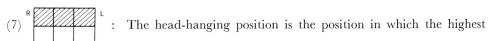 : These are called geotropic and apogeotropic

direction changing type of positional nystagmus.   They may be induced in cases with central lesions but are also seen sometimes with labyrinthine lesions.   Those from labyrinthine lesions usually have a rotating component and usually also are of short duration, i.e. disappear or change in a few days.

(6)   Spontaneous or positional nystagmus of labyrinthine origin is accompanied more or less by a sensation of vertigo.   The sensation of vertigo is usually parallel to the intensity of the nystagmus.   Very active spontaneous nystagmus of large amplitude without vertigo can always be regarded as being of central and not labyrinthine origin.

(7) 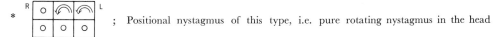 : The head-hanging position is the position in which the highest

incidence of positional nystagmus is evoked.   This is accordingly the head position which should be routinely examined and this position cannot be omitted in a screening examination.*

---

* R ☐ ◯ ⌒ ⌒ ☐ L
    ☐ ◯ ◯ ◯ ☐   ; Positional nystagmus of this type, i.e. pure rotating nystagmus in the head

hanging position and some others is frequently encountered in cases of paroxysmal positional vertigo. The utricle is known to mostly induce a rotating type of nystagmus when stimulated.   The pure rotating nystagmus which is encountered in head-hanging and some other positions is thus believed to be most likely of otolithic origin.

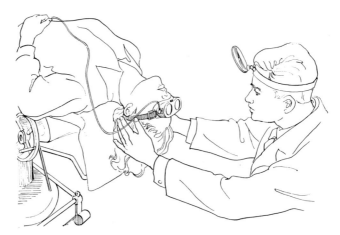

Fig. 17 Observation of eye movements behind Frenzel glasses in the head-hanging position.

d. Positioning nystagmus

Head position change is a routine part of daily life, although positions such as the head-hanging position are not usually assumed.

If vertigo was induced by the head position changes which are normally assumed during our daily life, or if nystagmus was provoked by head position alteration, our usual activities could not be easily accomplished. Positional or positioning nystagmus and/or vertigo are thus regarded as pathological.

Positional nystagmus is any persistent or long-lasting nystagmus which appears after the assumption of different head positions, while positioning nystagmus is any transitory nystagmus which appears directly after the head position changes. There may be a relatively long latency, several seconds or more, before nystagmus appears after positioning is completed.

Positioning nystagmus as well as positional nystagmus cannot be provoked in a subject with no labyrinth. Positioning nystagmus is believed to be initiated by the semicircular canals and probably also by the otolithic organs; it manifests itself in cases of both central and peripheral vestibular lesions.

Method. The test is performed with Frenzel glasses.

(1) The head position is changed from the sitting to the head-hanging position. The positioning is important since it frequently induces pure vertical nystagmus which signifies a central disturbance, and also induces pure rotating nystagmus which indicates a labyrinthine lesion (after STENGER, Fig. 18 a).

(2) The head position is changed from sitting to head hanging with the head twisted to the right or to the left. This positioning yields a high incidence of induced nystagmus (after DIX and HALLPIKE).

(3) The head is quickly twisted to the right or to the left in the supine position, and in the sitting position (Fig. 18 b). In the former, the positioning stimulates the otolithic organs and the lateral canals simultaneously, while in the latter it stimulates only the lateral canals.*

---

* In both of those, there are identical influences from neck torsion. To exclude these effects, positioning should be performed with the head and the body together. The influences from the neck are, however, usually small in the positioning nystagmus tests.

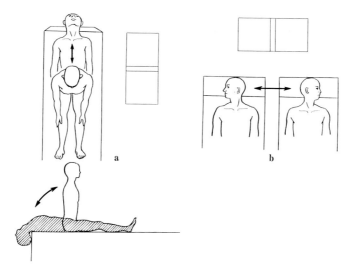

Fig. 18 Diagrams for recording positioning nystagmus and drawings indicating the corresponding head positions.
a: Head-body position change from the sitting to the head-hanging positions and vice versa.
   The position changes are performed in the sagittal as well as in the oblique planes.
b: Head position changes between two side head positions with the body supine.

Diagnostic Significance

(1)   The head position change from sitting to head-hanging along the sagittal plane
frequently provokes vertical nystagmus directed toward the chin.

When it is purely vertical, a central origin may be strongly suspected; especially when
it is of a large amplitude or long lasting, e.g., more than 10 seconds.   When the nystagmus
is of a small amplitude, the differentiation of purely vertical nystagmus from rotating-
vertical nystagmus is difficult: the latter can be peripheral in origin.   This indicates that
a small amplitude vertical nystagmus cannot be diagnosed as central or peripheral, i.e. a
final decision must be suspended.*

(2)   Vertical positioning of the head from sitting to head hanging may induce purely
vertical nystagmus directed towards the chin, and vertical positioning from the head-
hanging position induces pure vertical nystagmus directed towards the forehead.   This
is frequently found in degenerative diseases of the cerebellum, suggesting a defective
inhibitory mechanism.**

---

*   Vertical-rotating nystagmus directed downward   ⟨↓⟩   originates from the left anterior canal nerves,
and that directed upward ⟨↑⟩ originates from the left posterior canal nerve, when stimulated by electric
pulses.   Horizontal nystagmus originates from the lateral canal nerves.   When the three canal nerves
on the left side are simultaneously stimulated horizontal-rotating nystagmus or   ⟨↻→⟩   is induced.   Purely
vertical nystagmus directed downward ⟨↓⟩ can be induced by stimulation of the bilateral anterior canal nerves while that directed upward ⟨↑⟩ is induced from the bilateral posterior canal nerves. Purely
vertical nystagmus cannot be induced by electrically stimulating or destroying a unilateral labyrinth.

** Vertical positioning in specific cases can produce purely vertical nystagmus by stimulating the bilateral
vertical canals.   When only one labyrinth is functioning and the other side is "dead", purely vertical
positioning nystagmus can be produced by stimulating one vertical canal and inhibiting the other.
This does not happen, however, in normal subjects, probably because the effect of the stimulus which
would provoke vertical nystagmus is inhibited by central mechanisms which may be malfunctioning
during cerebellar disease.

(3)   Pure rotating nystagmus after head positioning is a very frequent finding in cases of paroxysmal positional vertigo.   The direction of rotation of the nystagmus is, in most instances, reversed when the direction of head positioning is reversed.

Identification of pure rotating nystagmus is best accomplished by observing the bulbar conjunctiva and not by observing the iris.   Identification of fine vertical nystagmus is also difficult because the eyelids move synchronously with nystagmus.   The differentiation of purely vertical nystagmus from rotating-vertical nystagmus is frequently difficult when the amplitude of the nystagmus is small.   If doubt exists about the eye movements observed, the best course is to strictly record the observations without attempting difficult interpretations.

3.   Significance of the Examination of Spontaneous, Positional and Positioning Nystagmus

The examination of spontaneous, positional and positioning nystagmus has basic importance for the whole equilibrium examination.   It should be compared with the examination of body equilibrium.   While eye movement reflex appears to be voluntary, it is actually largely controlled by CNS mechanisms, i.e. foveal-fixation reflex, vestibular reflex movements, brainstem reflexes etc.   Tiny changes in the CNS often influence eye movement.

The examination of eye movements may be divided into two parts: 1) the examination of gaze function (gaze nystagmus examination), or the examination of the mechanics of the laboratory balance and 2) the examination of the influence of changes in the CNS upon eye movements (non-gaze nystagmus examination) or the biasing of the balance. Although the vestibular system has strong external influences on the oculomotor system (Fig. 19), we should be aware of the varying origins of the abnormalities.   Spontaneous symptoms are of primary importance while some induced nystagmus evoked by head positioning, etc., should have a limited but specific diagnostic significance.

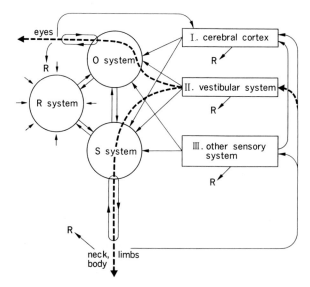

Fig. 19   Three major systems for equilibrium.
Oculomotor (O) and Spinal Motor Systems (S) are modulated by a Regulatory System(R).   These three major systems are further influenced from outside by three other systems; the cerebrocortical, the vestibular and other sensory inputs such as proprioception.

THE METHODS OF RECORDING OF EYE MOVEMENTS

1. The History of the Recording of Eye Movements

As indicated in the foregoing chapter, the careful observation of eye movements is helpful in the diagnosis and treatment of vestibular dysfunction. However, it became obvious many years ago that there was need of some more accurate system for measuring and recording eye movements. By the 1920's developments in the methods for recording eye movements were divided into two groups (after VERNON, 1928).

(1) The methods which depend upon direct photographs of the eye, of the reflection of light from the apex of the cornea, or from some small object attached to the cornea (DODGE and CLINE, 1902; COBURN, 1905; JUDD, et al., 1905; DOHLMAN, 1925; WIEDERSHEIM, 1931).

(2) The methods which depend upon the attachment of a capsule or recording lever to the cornea or eyelid.

(a) An air-filled sac may be placed tightly over the eyeball or the closed eye. Movements of the eye will then cause changes in the volume and pressure within the sac which may be recorded and correlated with eye movements (BUYS, 1909; WITMER, 1917).

(b) A recording lever may be attached to the eyeball or eyelid and the movements of this lever may be recorded by direct tracing on a kymograph (CORDS, 1927; OHM, 1928).

Although optical methods including the use of moving pictures (ASCHAN, 1958; GRAU and STROBEL, 1963) or television (see pages 66–67) may be still selected for recording certain eye movements, these two methods have been gradually superseded by electrical recordings of eye movements.

Initially SCHOTT (1922) used a string galvanometer for picking up the potential changes around the orbits induced by the movement of the eyes during nystagmus. The records thus obtained were thought to be generated by the action potentials of the extraocular muscles (MEYERS, 1929; JACOBSON, 1930). MOWRER et al. (1936), however, proved definitely that they were due to changes in the orientation of the standing potential between the cornea and retina which occurs during eye movements. The term electronystagmography (ENG), coined by MEYERS (1929), has been widely applied to this method as practiced by otologists. On the other hand, CARMICHAEL and DEARBORN (1947) introduced the term electro-oculography (EOG) to have a broader meaning of the recording of any eye movements including nystagmus.

FENN and HURSH (1937), HOFFMAN et al. (1939) and MILES (1939) studied the characteristics and determinants of the corneoretinal potential in detail. Clinical applications of ENG to analyses of physiological and pathological nystagmus were reported successively in 1939 by JUNG; JUNG and MITTERMAIER; PERLMAN and CASE; and LEKSELL. Furthermore, POWSNER and LION (1950) reported on the use of ENG in measuring the strength of the extraocular muscles. In 1951 TOROK et al. reported on a combination of optical and electrical methods utilizing a photoelectric cell which they named photoelectronystagmography.

There have been many developments during recent years in both research and clinical work in the recording of nystagmus. Notable among them are 1) an electrical devise designed by HENRIKSSON (1955a) for measuring the eye velocity of the slow phases of nystagmus which is based on principles similar to those described by POWSNER & LION (1950), and 2) the use of a direct current amplifier made possible by HALLPIKE et al. (1960) for the accurate recordings not only of nystagmic and other transient eye movements but also of sustained gaze deviation.

Comprehensive studies on the clinical application of the ENG were conducted by Aschan et al. (1956), Jongkees and Philipszoon (1964), Jung and Kornhuber (1964), and Kornhuber (1966).

2. Electronystagmography (ENG)
a. Principles (Fig. 20)

It is well known that a potential exists between the cornea and retina even when the eye is not illuminated (du Bois-Reymond, 1894). The cornea is positive relative to the retina and the standing corneo-retinal potential is about 1 millivolt in humans when measured by means of skin electrodes. "Thus the eyeball may be thought of as a rotatable battery situated within a conducting medium" (Marg, 1951).

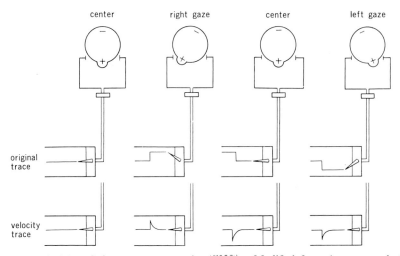

Fig. 20   The principles of electronystagmography (ENG).   Modified from Aschan et al. (1956).

If the electrodes are placed nasal and temporal to the right eye and the eyes are turned to the right, the temporal electrode will be much nearer the positive corneal pole and, conversely, the nasal electrode much nearer the negative or posterior pole, i.e. the retina. Thus the potential recorded between the electrodes changes with horizontal eye movement. If the eyes move upward or downward, similar potential changes can be picked up by placing the electrodes above and below the eyeball.

It may be realized that potential difference between any pair of electrodes situated around the orbit will not change during wheel rotations of the eyeball. Thus, rotary eye movements cannot be recorded by ENG.

ENG is thus defined as a method for recording eye movements by electronically amplifying and recording the potential changes accompanying eye movements.

b. Recording electrodes

i) Placement of electrodes.   Silver-silver chloride electrodes of disc-like shape with a diameter of 5 or 10 mm (similar to those used in E.E.G.) are used with conventional amplifiers, but special electrodes designed to minimize polarization are necessary for direct current amplifiers.

The position and number of electrodes is shown in Fig. 21. Namely, electrodes 1 and 2 for the temporal leads are placed on the horizontal line connecting both outer canthi, just outside of the external orbital margin of both the right and left eyes. No. 3 is at the bridge of the nose on the same horizontal line as are the bitemporal leads. Electrodes 4

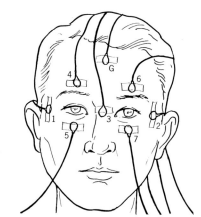

①-②: Bitemporal leads
①-③: Horizontal leads of the right eye
②-③: Horizontal leads of the left eye
④-⑤: Vertical leads of the right eye
⑥-⑦: Vertical leads of the left eye
  G: Ground electrode

Fig. 21 Standard electrode position for ENG.

and 5 are placed on the vertical line through the middle of the palpebral fissure of the right side, No. 4 being above the eyebrow and No. 5 below the inferior orbital margin. Electrodes 6 and 7 placed above and below the left eye correspond to Nos. 4 and 5 placed around the right eye. A ground electrode is located on the forehead.

The bitemporal (temporal-temporal) or temporal-nasal electrodes are used to record horizontal eye movements and the superior-inferior electrodes for vertical eye movements. Recording from the bitemporal pair gives an amplification effect of about two times that of the monocular pair. Therefore, in most cases in which both eyes perform associated movements during nystagmus, the bitemporal leads are preferable for recording horizontal eye movements.

After cleaning the skin with gauze soaked in benzine and applying electrode paste to the skin (volume equal to that of the electrode concave cavity) the electrode is fixed to the skin by means of plastic tape or bandage. The skin resistance of each pair is measured and recorded after placement of the electrodes. Values of interelectrode resistance below 20 kΩ are desirable, but not absolutely necessary in many cases.

Electric shielding is desirable to minimize inductive artifacts produced by A.C. current sources and to provide an electrically stabilized condition for the examination. In many cases, however, shielding is not indispensable for ENG recording.

ii) Adjustment of the amplifier. Usually an ink-writing polygraph is used for the ENG.

(1) Selection of the recording time constant (Fig. 22 A, B). The recording time constant is the time taken for the recorded potential to return to a level of $1/e$ of the input voltage applied continuously to the amplifier. Thus, if a steady or DC potential of 100μV is applied to an amplifier (input) and a time constant of 1.5 sec is selected, 1.5 sec is the time required for the amplifier potential (amplifier output) to decline to approximately one third of its original value, i.e. 37μV. With conventional ENG amplifiers various time constants may be selected.

It should be realized that the shorter the time constant, the greater the distortion of the record obtained; also the grade of distortion is greater as the potential changes become slower. However, if eye movements are recorded by a direct current amplifier, i.e. with a time constant equal to infinity, the tracings represent a direct record always in linear relation to the deviation of the eyes. If an alternating current amplifier with a relatively short time constant is used, the recording pen will return to the base line within a short period even though the eyes remain stationary in a certain position. (The

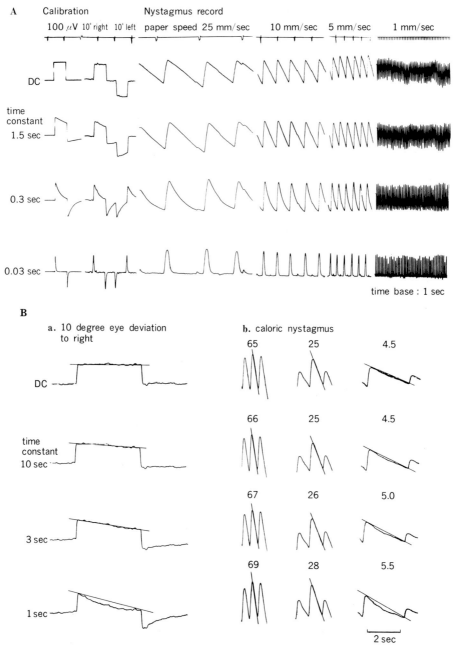

Fig. 22   A: Examples of calibration signals and eye movements recorded with different time constants. Lines 1, 2, 3, and 4 were recorded with DC and time constants of 1.5, 0.3 and 0.03 seconds respectively as labeled. Column 1 of lines 1–4 is a 100 μV calibration signal. Column 2 shows actual eye movements of 10° to the right and to the left.   Columns 3–6 are nystagmus recorded at various paper speeds as indicated by the time calibration (mm/sec) above each column.   The time mark is 1 sec.
B: Eye movements lines 1–4 recorded with DC and various time constants similar to A.   a: 10 degree eye deviation to the right.   b: Examples of caloric nystagmus of various intensity (slow phase velocity). Numbers in deg/sec above each trace indicate the slow phase velocity obtained by measuring the slopes of the nystagmus waves.   The most accurate velocities are obtained by measuring the D.C. recordings. Note that the error in velocity introduced by decreasing the recording time constant (lines 2, 3, 4) is magnified as the nystagmus becomes less intense.

record falsely indicates that the eyes have returned to their original position.) The speed for returning to the base line is, of course, faster, as the time constant is shortened.

In order to obtain records with the least distortion, direct current amplifiers or alternating current amplifiers with relatively long time constants should be used. In this case, however, the slow potential changes from physiological and nonphysiological sources are also faithfully recorded and base line fluctuation may be exaggerated. As accuracy and stability of routine tracings are not incompatible, a time constant should be chosen from within the allowable limits for recording relatively distortion-free nystagmus, but not so long as to allow the record to be affected by extraneous factors. For special purposes D. C. amplification, although sometimes troublesome, is preferred. Fig. 22 illustrates calibration and nystagmus records. With DC recording eye movements are faithfully recorded. Relatively long time constants of 3.0 and 1.5 seconds also produce records comparable to those of DC recordings but with short time constants of 0.3 and 0.03 seconds the record is seen to falsely return to the base line before the eyes have completed their movement to the midline position.

According to previous reports, the time constants used for ENG were 1.5 sec. (JUNG and TÖNNIES, 1948), 1.5–3.0 sec. (ASCHAN et al., 1955, 1956), 1.7 sec. (STAHLE, 1956), 2.0 sec. (PREBER, 1957), and 1.5 sec. (UEMURA, 1967). Records obtained with time constants of more than 1.0 sec. may be regarded as original traces of nystagmus.

On the other hand, if recordings are made with time constants shorter than 0.05 seconds, the pen deflects only during the eye movement and in the "differentiated record" thus obtained, the amplitude of the pen deflection is proportional to the velocity of the eye movement but not to its magnitude (HENRIKSSON, 1955a). Therefore the velocity of eye movement may be directly recorded. The tracings thus obtained are designated as velocity traces of nystagmus.

(2) Determination of amplification. Initially, the amplification is adjusted so that an input voltage of 100 microvolts will give a pen deflection of 10 mm. With this amplification (bitemporal recording) a horizontal deviation of 10 degrees produces pen deflections ranging from 10 to 30 mm in normal subjects.

The maximum amplitude of nystagmus which will be recorded should remain within the limits of the pen deflection. Since a nystagmus amplitude greater than 20 degrees only rarely appears in experimentally induced nystagmus, we have found that an amplification of 10 to 15 mm for a 10 degree eye deviation is usually optimal.

(3) Paper speed. The standard speed for recording is usually 10 mm per second; this is convenient for quantitative analysis of tracings.

Different paper speeds also are recommended for specific purposes; 5 mm/sec for surveying the entire course of caloric nystagmic reaction (HENRIKSSON, 1955a) and 1 mm/sec for observing optokinetic responses as a pattern (SUZUKI and KOMATSUZAKI, 1962).

iii) Calibration procedure. Calibration is performed by having the subject look at small electric lights placed straight ahead, 10 degrees to the right, left, up and down respectively (Fig. 23). The polarities are adjusted as follows; in the horizontal leads an eye movement to the right causes an upward deflection of the recording pen and a movement to the left a downward deflection. In vertical leads an upward eye movement is recorded as an upward deflection of the pen and vice versa.

The calibration procedure should be performed at the start and at the end of each recording. If there is any difference between the calibrations, the values which were obtained at the time nearer to the point of measurement should be applied.

For the calibration of eye speed it is most convenient to use constant velocity triangle

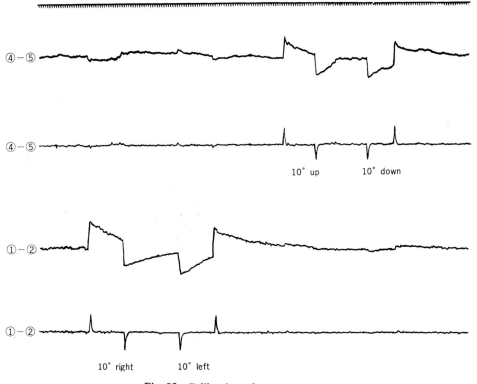

Fig. 23 Calibration of eye movements.
The numbers at the left side of ENG traces indicate those of electrodes as seen in Fig. 21; ①–② are the bitemporal leads and ④–⑤ the vertical leads of the right eye. This convention is to be applied to all succeeding ENG traces. In each pair the upper record is a tracing obtained with a time constant of 1.5 seconds and the lower record with a time constant of 0.03 seconds. The time base is shown above at 10 marks per second.

waves. Initially the 10 degree calibration is carried out (Fig. 24A) and a certain amplitude of pen deflection is obtained on the original eye movement tracings (*a* mm in Fig. 24A). Next, without changing the amplification, triangle waves of a certain input voltage with a frequency of 0.5 cycle per second are substituted for the eye movement. At that time their input voltage is adjusted by a potentiometer to give the same amplitude as a 10 degree eye deviation (Fig. 24B). The pen deflection on the eye speed tracings thereby obtained (*b* mm in Fig. 24B) corresponds to two times the eye speed of 10 degrees per sec., i.e. 20 degrees per sec.; if the pen deflections are electronically clipped in one direction, an eye speed of 10 degrees per sec. is then equal to the amplitude of pen deflection.

   c. **Findings appearing on the ENG**
   i) *Nystagmus.* Nystagmus has been classified into two types by subjective observation, i.e. jerking and pendular nystagmus; other types seen less frequently are pendular jerk and "hüpfender Nystagmus" (FRENZEL, 1942) or "Spitzennystagmus" (JUNG, 1953).

   According to the wave shapes recorded with the ENG the nystagmus which was observed to be pendular can be further classified into various forms of sine waves, saw-tooth waves or their intermediate variations. The nystagmus which appeared to be jerking also represents a variety of forms other than the typical oscillations consisting of combinations of the slow and quick phases. Moreover, a type of record in which two different shapes

A. 10 degree calibration   **B. triangle waves of 0.5 cycle per second**

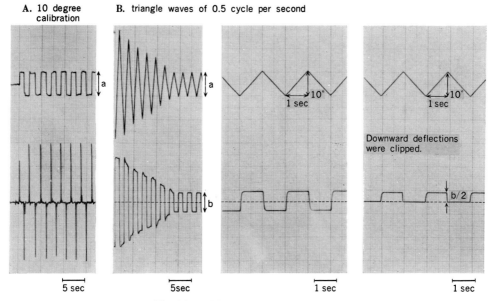

Fig. 24   Calibration of eye velocity.

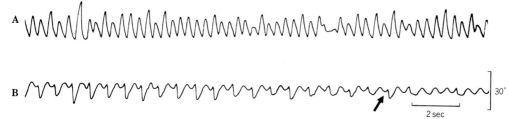

Fig. 25   Caloric nystagmus in a case of congenital nystagmus recorded with the eyes open in light. The upper trace shows the summation of congenital pendular nystagmus and calorically induced nystagmus toward the right(A) and the lower the superimposition of pendular nystagmus and caloric nystagmus towards the left(B).   The arrow indicates the termination of caloric nystagmus and thereafter congenital nystagmus only was present.   Generally, there is no superimposition of spontaneous vestibular nystagmus and induced vestibular nystagmus.

of pendular and jerking nystagmus are superimposed upon each other has been obtained (Fig. 25).

In addition to qualitative analysis of the wave forms, ENG has made it possible to analyze the fine details of induced nystagmus such as its onset, frequency, amplitude, velocity of slow and quick phases, and termination.

ii)   Eye movements other than nystagmus

(1)   Pendular eye movements.   Slow waves of high amplitude with a frequency of 0.3 per second occur in normal subjects during eye closure while tired or sleepy.   It was noted, however, that similar waves are often present in post-traumatic patients especially those with cerebral concussion (ADAMS and STAEWEN, 1959; LANGE and KORNHUBER, 1962).

(2)   Square wave jerks.   Square waves with a frequency of about 2 per second and amplitude from 2 to 10 degrees may be recorded in normal persons (JUNG and KORNHUBER, 1964) and more frequently in senile patients with cerebral arteriosclerosis.   Similar to and fro movements showing a crenelated shape on ENG were also observed after a vertigi-

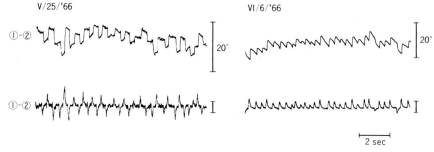

Fig. 26 Transition from square wave jerks to spontaneous nystagmus.
The records were obtained from the same patient at an interval of 11 days with eye closed on both occasions. In each pair the upper tracing was obtained with a time constant of 1.5 seconds and the lower with a time constant of 0.05 seconds. The calibrations for the lower traces are 100°/sec.

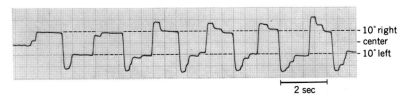

Fig. 27 Ocular dysmetria seen in a case with a cerebellar hemisphere cyst extending to the midline (DC recording).
The patient was asked to look alternately at each of two targets 20 degrees apart in the horizontal plane. The overshoot of the eyes on attempted fixation was present to either side but was most prominent on looking to the left. The initial overshoot to the left was corrected by three small saccades to the right.

nous attack as a transitional wave form from spontaneous nystagmus to square wave jerks (Fig. 26).

Abnormal high amplitude square waves 20 to 50 degrees usually with a frequency of 1 to 3 per second occurring during eye closure were rarely found as a sequel to brainstem encephalitis or pontocerebellar atrophy (Jung and Kornhuber, 1964).

(3) Ocular dysmetria, flutter-like oscillations of the eyes and opsoclonus. According to Cogan (1954), ocular dysmetria is an abnormality of eye movement analogous to the dysmetria of the limbs of cerebellar origin, in which a movement is performed with characteristic over- or undershooting and a lack of precision (Fig. 27). Flutter-like oscillations refer to the occurrence of intermittent to and fro oscillations of the eyes during fixation and saccadic movements. These movements are associated with disease of the cerebellum and cerebellar pathways. The duration of the oscillations is 0.3 to 1.0 seconds, the frequency 8 to 10 per second, and the amplitude approximately 5 to 10 degrees (Goldberg and Jampel, 1963).

Opsoclonus is the name applied by Orzechowski (1927) to the ocular movements described as an ocular hyperkinesia because of the alleged similarity to myoclonus in the peripheral motor system. This abnormality can be distinguished from flutter-like oscillations in that opsoclonus occurs in all planes, though mainly in the horizontal, lasts for more than 2 to 3 seconds and has a frequency of up to 13 per second and an irregularly varying amplitude of 2 to 40 degrees. Unlike ocular dysmetria and flutter it is not necessarily indicative of cerebellar disease but may be related to brainstem encephalitis.

Atkin and Bender (1964) also reported a variety of ocular myoclonus which they called lightning eye movements. These consist of occasional short bursts of rapid conjugate to and fro horizontal eye movements often following certain changes in gaze direction.

ENG recording revealed in most cases that each burst, usually 3–5 degrees in amplitude, lasts less than 0.5 second and contains 3 or 4 movements with a frequency of about 6–8 per second. A tegmental-pretectal lesion of the midbrain was considered to play an important role in the occurrence of this abnormality.

Because of certain similarities of opsoclonus, ocular flutter and ocular dysmetria (especially between the first two), it was postulated that opsoclonus represents a more severe and extensive disturbance, while ocular flutter is only a milder varient of opsoclonus (DYKEN and KOLÁŘ, 1968). However, since differentiation between these phenomena can be made more definitely with the use of ENG, it is preferable to deal with them separately.

iii) Wave forms which should be differentiated from nystagmus or abnormal eye movements

ENG can record many potential changes such as brain waves, muscle potentials, cardiac potential changes and others not related to eye movements.* They are, however, easily distinguished with a little experience because of their lower amplitude and characteristic differences from the potentials caused by eye movement or nystagmus.

An error in identification may arise from large amplitude waves accompanying blinking movements. Involuntary blinking movements appear as upward spikes of high amplitude in the vertical leads and are scarcely recorded in the horizontal leads in most cases (see Fig. 29a). If blinks produce small waves in the horizontal leads, their acutely angled spikes are easily distinguished from the more rectangle-like spikes of nystagmus. Recording with a time constant of less than 0.1 second makes their differentiation difficult.

Lid nystagmus (ADAMS, 1957) is defined as nystagmus occurring in the horizontal plane synchronously with blinks. Each horizontal beat has a longer duration than that of each blink recorded in the vertical leads (Fig. 29b).

Thus, when using a time constant of more than 1.0 second, blinks can be distinguished from nystagmus by their wave shapes or by the indication of blinks in the vertical leads. Blinking is not completely under voluntary control. Asking the patient not to blink often only increases the amount of blinking.

The discrimination of nystagmus from lid movement during eye closure is not as easy as it is when the eyes are open (Fig. 29c). A spasm of the eyelid sometimes causes nystagmus-like waves, but even in this case there are still several distinguishing features;

---

* When the corneoretinal potential is lost following disease or trauma of the eye as well as enucleation of the eyeball or when the eyeball is immobile, monocular recording of the affected side may pick up the potential change accompanied by eye movements of the intact side and reveal small reverse-shape spikes (Fig. 28).

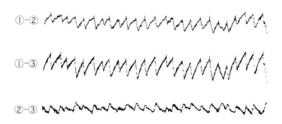

Fig. 28 Apparent dissociated nystagmus due to loss of the corneoretinal potential in the left eye (②–③).
Caloric nystagmus toward the left was observed equally in both eyes by direct observation. Note the smaller amplitude in the bitemporal leads (①–②) than in the monocular leads of the right eye (①–③). The traces were recorded with similar amplification of 10mm for 100μV.

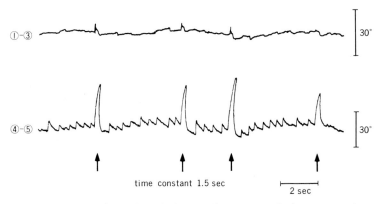

Fig. 29 a Blinks (↑) and vertical upward nystagmus during eye opening.

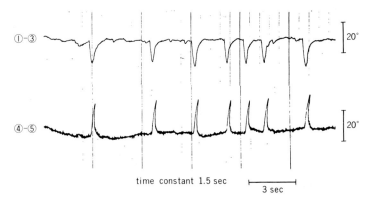

Fig. 29 b Lid nystagmus seen in a case with pinealoma.
Nystagmus toward the left was recorded through the horizontal leads of the right eye (①–③) synchronously with the spikes caused by blinks in the vertical leads of the same eye (④–⑤). Note a longer duration of the nystagmus spike than of the blinking movement.

relatively symmetrical ascending and descending wave shapes are quite different from those of the quick and slow phases of nystagmus; the appearance of these spasms becomes less frequent as the recording continues; and these waves may disappear when the examiner lightly places his finger on the closed lid (Fig. 29d). In order to avoid confusion in identifying nystagmus, the recording of eye closure is not recommended for tests inducing vertical nystagmus, such as the positioning nystagmus test (according to STENGER, 1955).

The advantages of recording nystagmus or abnormal eye movements by means of ENG can be summarized as follows.

(1)   Since permanent graphic records of eye movements including nystagmus are obtained by ENG, exact analysis and objective comparison of the test results performed at various times can be made during the course of any disease.

(2)   The quantitative analysis of nystagmus as regards its amplitude, frequency, and eye speed of the slow and quick phases, and qualitative analysis of the wave forms of nystagmus or abnormal eye movements were made possible by the use of ENG. This results in raising the accuracy of the diagnostic evaluation of nystagmus and abnormal eye movements.

(3)   ENG can record eye movements not only with the eyes open in light but also with

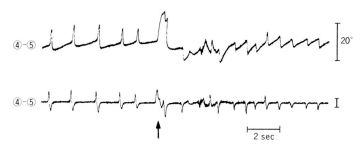

Fig. 29 c Spasm of the eyelid and vertical nystagmus.
In the supine position the spikes were solely recorded synchronously with eyelid spasm while vertical downward nystagmus appeared after the patient was placed in a left side down position (arrow). The upper trace was recorded with a 1.5 second time constant and the lower traced with a 0.05 second time constant. The calibration for the lower trace is 100°/sec. Note the difference in the wave form between the spikes.

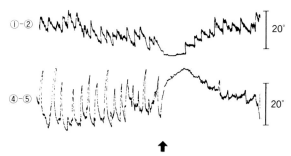

Fig. 29 d The effect of pressure on the eyelid to lid spasm and nystagmus.
The vertical spikes (④–⑤) produced by eyelid spasm disappeared after the examiner lightly placed his finger on the closed lid (arrow), but horizontal nystagmus recorded in the bitemporal leads (①–②) remained unchanged.

the eyes open in darkness or closed. Recording in darkness or with the eyes closed was impossible prior to the advent of the ENG. Recording eye movements in the dark (no visual fixation) often reveals nystagmus which is not seen by means of direct observation of the eyes open in light. Also, the comparison of ocular findings obtained under several different conditions of light and fixation may provide information useful in clarifying the origin of nystagmus.

On the other hand, ENG has the disadvantage that rotatory eye movements cannot be recorded with this method, as they cause no corneoretinal potential shift. In addition, there are instrumental limitations such as the distortion of records by using an AC amplifier or the sensitivity of the instrument to various extraneous potentials and artefacts.

Thus, it must be kept in mind that the use of ENG does not necessarily predicate perfect recording of ocular findings, and that a comparison of the ENG with direct visual observation of eye movements will be inevitably necessary for discussing their diagnostic significance.

d. Standard procedure of ENG in the spontaneous nystagmus test and positional and positioning tests

In order to provide an adequate examination and permanent record, the recordings of spontaneous and provoked nystagmus by means of ENG are routinely performed as follows. Simultaneous recordings of horizontal eye movements through the bitemporal leads and of vertical eye movements through the vertical leads of either right or left eye are required.

Spontaneous nystagmus tests: After calibrating with gaze movements to the right, left, up and down as described in the foregoing chapter, the patient is asked to look at a point in the ceiling directly in the midline of his visual field. After continuous recording in this visual fixation condition for 30 seconds, the patient is asked to close his eyes and then the room lights are turned off. The eyes remain closed for 30 seconds, and then the patient is asked to do a mental calculation with his eyes still closed and the recording is continued for another 20 seconds. Goggles covered with black paper in order to completely eliminate light are placed on the subject's eyes. About 20 seconds later the patient is asked to open his eyes. This corresponds to the condition of eyes open in darkness and the recording is continued for another 30 seconds.

Nystagmus demonstrated under these three different conditions (eyes open in light, eyes closed and eyes open in darkness) by the procedure described above has raised the percentage of detected pathologic nystagmus and has also been helpful in topical diagnosis.

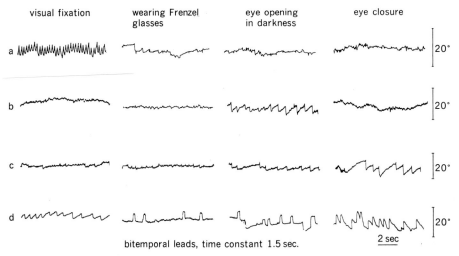

Fig. 30 Variation of nystagmus under different visual conditions.
Congenital nystagmus, which was prominent when the patient fixated in the light, could hardly be recognized under conditions other than those of visual fixation (Case a). Although in cases of Ménière's disease nystagmus was not manifest upon visual fixation, jerking nystagmus was recorded exclusively in the non-fixated condition, for example eye open in darkness (Case b) and eyes closed (Case c). On the other hand, in certain cases with brainstem lesions there are different findings under the various conditions of visual fixation, eyes open in darkness and eyes closed as in Case d. This modification of nystagmus is not seen with peripheral lesions of the labyrinth or VIIIth nerve.

The results of spontaneous nystagmus tests in several cases with spontaneous nystagmus of various origins are shown in Fig. 30. In two cases of Ménière's disease, i.e. Cases b and c, visual fixation in the light or wearing Frenzel glasses did not reveal any nystagmus. However, nystagmus became manifest in Case b, when the eyes were opened in darkness and in Case c during eye closure. Congenital nystagmus, conversely, often disappeared under these special conditions (Case a), and nystagmus of central origin could be modified by these special conditions (Case d). Case d is further described in the chapter of Case Studies (Case 8). Furthermore, Fig. 31 demonstrates a variety of spontaneous nystagmus under different visual conditions including the change of gaze direction in the light.

Non-specific provocation such as loading by a mental calculation or talking to the patient can often reveal pathological nystagmus and make obscure nystagmus manifest; it is an important procedure in the recording of nystagmus.

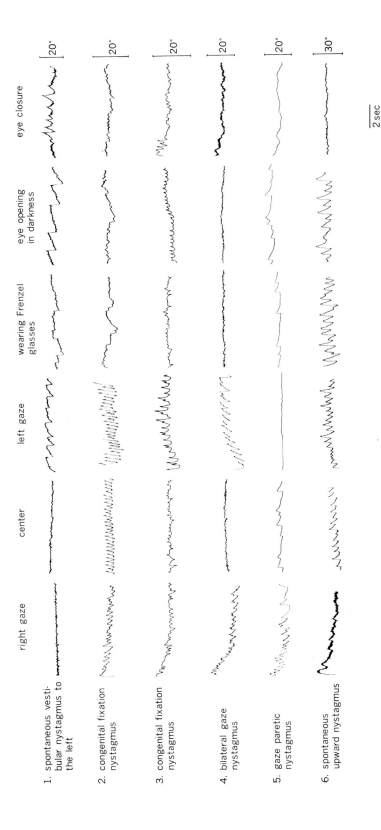

Fig. 31 A variety of spontaneous nystagmus recorded under different visual conditions.

The five traces from the top to the fifth were recorded with a 1.5 second time constant through horizontal leads and the sixth through vertical leads. This figure is similar to Fig. 30 except that the recordings shown are expanded to include different gaze conditions in the light.

Positional and positioning tests: The above mentioned spontaneous nystagmus tests are then followed by the positional test and the positioning test.

The positional test: While the patient is lying in the supine position he is asked and helped to turn his head and body slowly first to the right side and then back to the supine position.   Next he turns to the left lateral position and then back to the supine position. Each lateral position is maintained for one minute.

The positioning test: Following the positional test, the positioning test is performed by bringing the patient from the sitting position rapidly to a supine position with the head hanging back for about 30 seconds and subsequently rapidly back to the sitting position.

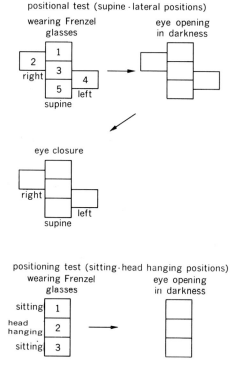

Fig. 32   Diagram of the positoinal and positioning tests to be used with ENG recording.
The block diagrams illustrate the position and the order of the postural change. The standard positions indicated have been previously described (see Fig. 16). In addition it is recommended that the order of change of position be performed sequentially as indicated by the numbers 1–5 and 1–3 under each of the different visual conditions.

These tests are performed under the three different conditions of wearing Frenzel glasses, eyes open in darkness and eyes closed as shown in Fig. 32.   The appearance and changes in the character of nystagmus should be examined.   Positional and positioning tests as "provoked nystagmus tests" should be included in the tests using ENG together with the spontaneous nystagmus tests.   In these tests both horizontal and vertical leads should be recorded simultaneously with two amplifiers for each direction, one for the original traces and one for the velocity traces.

The necessity for applying simultaneous recording of horizontal and vertical leads cannot be overemphasized in that the direction, toward which the nystagmus will appear, cannot be predicted.   Also by recording velocity traces as well as original traces for each direction the blanks in the original traces which may occur momentarily after posture changes will be compensated for by the findings obtained from the velocity traces (Fig. 33). Therefore ENG recording of positional and positioning tests cannot be sufficiently performed by means of a two-channel polygraph; 4 channels are necessary.

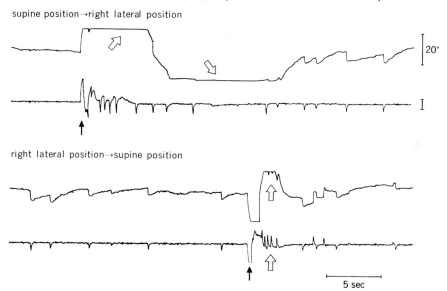

Fig. 33 Overexcursion of the recording pen following the postural changes.
The loss of information about eye movements in the original traces (upper traces) due to overexcursion of the pen immediately after posture changes (arrows) may be partially compensated for by the velocity traces (lower traces). Since the velocity trace has a shorter recording time constant (0.05 second) when compared to the time constant of the original trace (1.5 second), the velocity trace shows a more rapid recovery after overloading. During the time of overload of the original traces indicated by the hollow arrows the velocity traces show that some nystagmus was occurring. The calibration for the velocity traces is 100°/sec.

The findings obtained from the positional and positioning tests using ENG are classified as follows and are indicated in Figs. 34–40.

1) Nystagmus provoked solely by rapid posture change (Fig. 34).

Nystagmus appears for less than 10 seconds after rapidly assuming a lateral position or reassuming the supine position, and its direction corresponds to that of post-rotatory nystagmus.

2) Spontaneous nystagmus provoked by posture change (Fig. 35).

A nystagmus, not found in the supine position, may appear for the first time with a change in posture. Its strength is maximum immediately after the new position is reached, and it disappears or definitely lessens within about 30 seconds if there is no further change of position.

3) Spontaneous nystagmus influenced by posture change (Fig. 36).

A nystagmus previously present in the supine position is strengthened with a change in posture; its strength is maintained constant after returning to the original supine position. From this feature spontaneous nystagmus can be differentiated from a directionfixed positional nystagmus. Compare Figs. 36 and 37 described below.

4) Direction-fixed positional nystagmus (Fig. 37).

A nystagmus first occurs (Fig. 37a) or is strengthened (Fig. 37b) with a change in position, and persists for more than 30 seconds as long as the new position is maintained.

rapid change from the left lateral
to the supine position

slow change from the left lateral
to the supine position

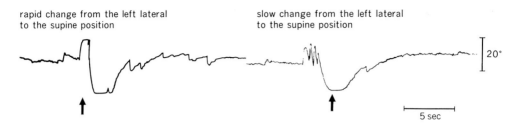

20°

5 sec

Fig. 34 Nystagmus provoked solely by rapid posture change.
In this and the subsequent six figures arrows indicate posture change. The records in Fig. 34–40 were obtained with a 1.5 second time constant.

supine position → left lateral position

left lateral position → supine position

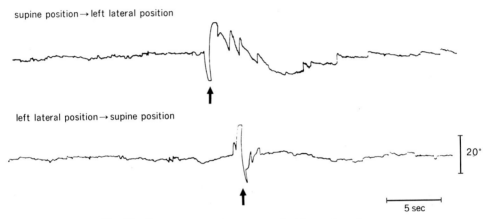

20°

5 sec

Fig. 35 Spontaneous nystagmus provoked by posture change.

supine position → left lateral position

left lateral position → supine position

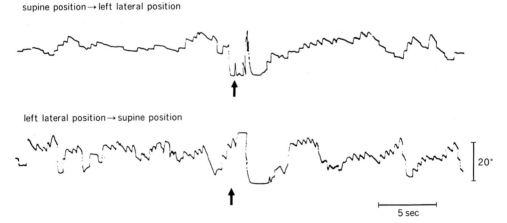

20°

5 sec

Fig. 36 Spontaneous nystagmus influenced by posture change.
Nystagmus was accentuated in the left lateral position but remained unchanged when the supine position was reassumed.

After returning to the supine position, the nystagmus disappears (Fig. 37a) or is reduced to its original intensity (Fig. 37b).

5) Direction-changing positional nystagmus (Fig. 38).

When assuming the left or right lateral position, a nystagmus, whose direction is opposite to that present in the supine or another lateral position, persistently occurrs

supine position → left lateral position

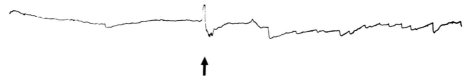

left lateral position → supine position

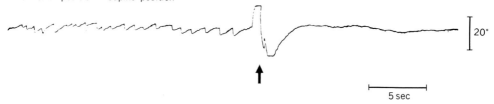

20°

5 sec

a. Nystagmus first appeared in the left lateral position and disappeared when the supine position was reassumed.

supine position → right lateral position

right lateral position → supine position

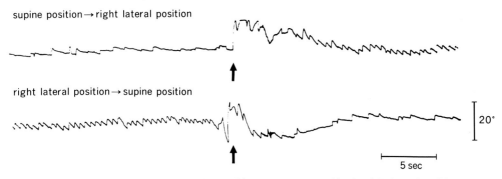

20°

5 sec

b. Nystagmus already present in the supine position was accentuated in the right lateral position and returned to the original strength when the supine position was reassumed.

Fig. 37 Direction-fixed positional nystagmus.

supine position → left lateral position

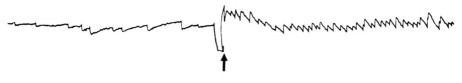

left lateral position → supine position

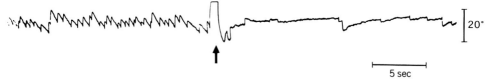

20°

5 sec

Fig. 38 Direction-changing positional nystagmus.

supine position → right lateral position

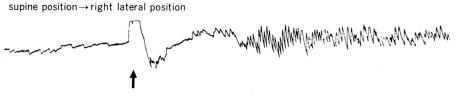

right lateral position → supine position

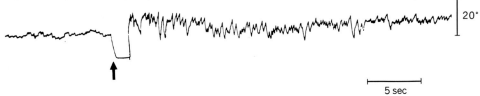

20°

5 sec

Fig. 39 Horizontal positioning nystagmus with "Gegenläufigkeit."

sitting position → head hanging position

head hanging position → sitting position

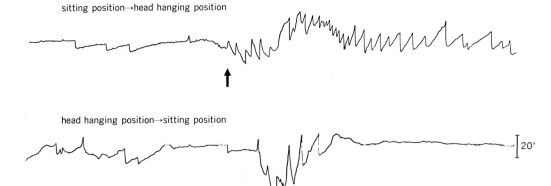

20°

3 sec

Fig. 40 Vertical positioning nystagmus.

(→ → ← or ○ → ←). According to FRENZEL (1955), this positional nystagmus can be further divided into irregular or regular type, depending upon whether or not nystagmus is present in the supine position (← ← → irregular, ← ○ → regular).

6) Horizontal positioning nystagmus (Fig. 39).

A transitory horizontal nystagmus may occur when the position is changed from the supine to the right or left lateral position, or when changed from the sitting to the head hanging position. It usually reaches a peak in several seconds and gradually recedes or disappears. Returning to the supine or sitting position is sometimes accompanied by a transitory nystagmus directed to the opposite side (GEGENLÄUFIGKEIT–STENGER, 1955).

7) Vertical positioning nystagmus (Fig. 40).

A transitory vertical nystagmus with similar character to that in 6) or with peak strength immediately after brought to the head hanging position may be induced by the positioning test. In some instances reversal of the nystagmus direction is also noted when the patient is brought back to the sitting position.

Recording ENG in the positional and positioning tests makes it possible to obtain objective information regarding the onset of the nystagmus and any alteration of its

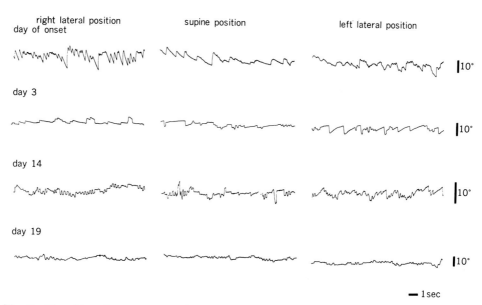

right lateral position
day of onset   supine position   left lateral position

day 3

day 14

day 19

— 1 sec

Fig. 41   Transition of nystagmus type during the course of right-sided Ménière's disease in a 40 year-old female.

All records were taken with the eyes open in darkness. On the day of onset the nystagmus to the right was revealed in the supine, right and left lateral positions (spontaneous nystagmus directed to the affected side). Three days later the direction of nystagmus in the left lateral position has changed to the left (divergent direction-changing positional nystagmus). Fourteen days later nystagmus to the left only was present in the supine and left lateral positions (spontaneous nystagmus directed to the unaffected side). No nystagmus was evident after 19 days.

character. In addition it is useful to differentiate positional and positioning nystagmus from spontaneous nystagmus and further classify each of them into subgroups. Since kinetic influences may be more or less pronounced even though a new position is slowly assumed, it can not be certainly stated that any nystagmus appearing in the positional test is solely due to static effects accompanying the change of posture. Thus we prefer to divide positional and positioning nystagmus by means of the character of the nystagmus, as mentioned above. The diagnostic evaluation of positional and positioning nystagmus thus subdivided remains an unsolved problem for future investigation.

One of the reasons for this obscurity seems to be that changes in the features of positional and positioning nystagmus during the course of a disease have been disregarded for a long time. Repetitive examinations of cases with unilateral labyrinthine lesions, including Ménière's disease, aural vertigo of unknown etiology and sudden deafness, afford sufficient evidence that after an acute episode the characteristics of nystagmus may vary.

A typical case is illustrated in Fig. 41; (day of onset) spontaneous nystagmus directed to the affected side, (day 3) divergent direction-changing positional nystagmus, (day 14) spontaneous nystagmus to the unaffected side. Although this case showed no nystagmus at day 19, some other cases demonstrated a convergent direction-changing positional nystagmus about 2–3 weeks after the acute episode (see Fig. 117).

Therefore, a difference in the type of positional or positioning nystagmus does not necessarily depend on a different location of the lesion, and features other than the direction of nystagmus are necessary for the classification essential to topographic evaluation.

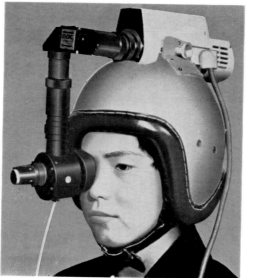
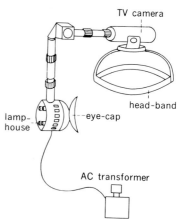

Fig. 43 TV oculoscope.

TESTS FOR SEMICIRCULAR CANAL FUNCTION

1. The Caloric Test

The caloric test is the method for examining the reactions induced by thermal stimulation of the labyrinth. It has the advantage that each labyrinth can be tested individually. When the caloric reaction is markedly depressed or absent, it provides one clear proof of a labyrinthine or vestibular nerve lesion on the stimulated side. The rotation test conversely stimulates both labyrinths simultaneously, and it is often difficult to determine the side of the defect if any is present.

On the other hand, although the angular acceleration in the rotation test acts directly on the cupular mechanism, thermal stimuli must be transmitted from the external auditory meatus to the labyrinth, where they are transformed into the appropriate modality to activate the semicircular canals. Because this mode of stimulation is indirect, the evoked effects are subject to much individual variation.

Among the numerous theories concerning the mechanism of the caloric stimulation of the labyrinth, BÁRÁNY's view that convection currents of the endolymph are induced within the semicircular canals and produce deflection of the cupula was confirmed by experimental studies (MAIER and LION, 1921; MEURMAN, 1924; DOHLMAN, 1925; SCHMALTZ, 1932; STEINHAUSEN, 1933).

In patients with Ménière's disease CAWTHORNE and COBB (1954) demonstrated that, on irrigation of the external auditory meatus with water above or below body temperature, a significant portion of the thermal change thus induced was transmitted to the perilymphatic space of the lateral semicircular canal. After inserting two thermocouples in the bony lateral semicircular canal a centimeter apart, they found a definite difference in temperature between the two after caloric stimulation.

Eye movements induced by vestibular stimulation provide a convenient parameter of labyrinthine reaction. In this regard, it was noted recently that the time course of the eye speed of the slow phase of nystagmus induced by caloric stimulation is well correlated to the strength of stimulation and can be divided into three parts as shown in Fig. 44 (Van EGMOND and TOLK, 1954).

In the first part, as the change in temperature is spreading through the bony semicircular canals to the endolymph, the eye speed gradually increases, until a temperature balance is attained. This balance is reached in the second part of the graph and the eye speed remains constant for this period. The maximum slow phase eye speed during this period depends on the temperature of water and the duration of this period at the maximum velocity depends on the duration of irrigation. After cessation of irrigation, as seen in the third part of the graph, the eye speed gradually decreases in parallel with the decrease in the temperature differential.

Viewed from the close relationship between the eye speed of the slow phase of nystagmus and the cupula deviation, Fig. 44 should represent a real picture of the cupula deviation after irrigation.

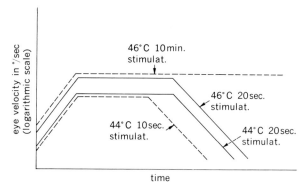

Fig. 44 The time course of the eye speed of the slow phase of nystagmus induced by different caloric stimuli (Van EGMOND and TOLK, 1954).
The ordinate is slow phase speed plotted on a logarithmic scale and the abscissa is time. Irrigation was performed with 44 °C and 46 °C water for different periods of time. Note that the maximum slow phase eye speed is solely dependent upon the temperature of the irrigating solution once the equilibrium condition is reached. The duration of nystagmus is related to the period of irrigation. Further explanation is in the text.

a. Methods of examination

Since BÁRÁNY (1906) first introduced caloric stimulation of the labyrinth into clinical practice as a labyrinthine function test, innumerable methods have been described. Among the variables in the testing method, the temperature of the water and the duration of stimulation as well as the method of measuring the response must be considered. A standard method for this test has not yet been established.

If complete results are to be obtained by caloric testing, the combination of cold and hot irrigations is necessary, as not only a hypoexcitability of one labyrinth but also a directional preponderance of induced nystagmus can be detected (as later described). Also the mass irrigation method has the advantage that the temperature of water reached can be adjusted accurately and well maintained at a certain degree. From these points of view, there seems to be no objection to the view of FITZGERALD and HALLPIKE (1942) that the alternate cold and hot caloric test enables one to push to its limits the resolving power of the caloric test.

Although a directional preponderance may be revealed by the caloric test, this does not mean that this finding belongs to caloric testing exclusively, as it can be revealed more clearly by means of other examinations. Consequently, if the purpose of caloric test is limited to detecting a hypoexcitability of the labyrinth, the test may be simplified as follows.

i) Simple caloric test

The patient should be supine with his head on a pillow to elevate it 30 degrees above the horizontal in order to bring the lateral semicircular canal into the true vertical plane.

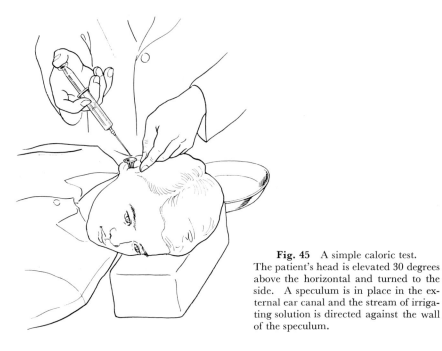

Fig. 45 A simple caloric test. The patient's head is elevated 30 degrees above the horizontal and turned to the side. A speculum is in place in the external ear canal and the stream of irrigating solution is directed against the wall of the speculum.

The patient's head is then turned with the tested ear upwards (Fig. 45).   20 °C water is drawn into a 5 ml syringe with a 20-gauge needle and introduced into the external meatus through the ear speculum in such a way that the stream is directed against the wall of the speculum, until the meatus is completely filled with the water.   The speculum should be the largest which will fit into the meatus.   A stop watch is started at the beginning of irrigation.

After keeping the patient in this position for 20 seconds, his head is brought back slowly to face the ceiling and Frenzel glasses are placed over his eyes.   Nystagmus is then observed in a semi-darkened room and the end point of nystagmus is measured from the start of irrigation.

When a perforation in the tympanic membrane is present, a solution of antibiotics may be injected into the ear in the same way as described above to avoid resulting infection.

The strength of 20 °C stimulation for 20 seconds roughly corresponds to that of 30 °C stimulation for 40 seconds.   Nystagmus lasts about two minutes in normal subjects and the difference in nystagmus duration between both labyrinths should not exceed 20 seconds. On evaluation of the simple caloric test, however, significance should only be attached to a definitely weak reaction lasting for less than 90 seconds.   Such a response is judged as a moderate hypoexcitability (canal paresis) of the tested labyrinth.   If no nystagmus is induced with 20 °C water, the test is repeated with 10 °C water.   Lack of response at this point indicates a severe or complete impairment of labyrinthine function.

Dix and Hallpike (1952) divided the test results in accordance with the following nomenclature: (1) Complete canal paresis.   No response obtained with irrigation at 20 °C for one minute. (2) Severe canal paresis.   No response obtained with stimuli of normal strength, i.e. 30 °C or 44 °C for 40 seconds; a response, however, was obtained with water at 20 °C for one minute.   (3) Moderate canal paresis.   In this group, responses, although obviously reduced, were obtained with stimuli of normal strength.

Whether complete canal paresis in the caloric test always means a dead labyrinth is questionable, as paralytic nystagmus to the intact side may be induced after the labyrinth with complete canal paresis has been surgically destroyed.

In addition to being simple to perform, seldom disturbing the patient by nausea or severe vertigo, and producing nystagmus easy to observe, there are several other advantages of the simple test. Water of 20 °C is easily prepared and stable (close to room temperature), the application of stimulus is not elaborate because of the procedure of filling the meatus with water and only one variable, the end point of induced nystagmus is measured. If more detailed information is desired, the nystagmus induced by caloric stimulation may be recorded with ENG during eye opening in darkness.

A simple comparison between the right and left ears may not be useful for interpretation of the test results, though a difference of more than 20 seconds is taken as being abnormal. Such difference may be caused either from a hypoexcitability of one labyrinth (or hyperexcitability of the other side), or from a directional preponderance in nystagmus to one direction. Furthermore, when the difference between both sides does not exceed 20 seconds, the result cannot invariably be regarded as normal; i.e. there is a possibility that the difference in the cold water irrigation will diminish to within the normal limit of 20 seconds, if a hypoexcitability of one labyrinth is combined with a directional preponderance to the other side as shown in Fig. 48 d.

Therefore, it must be kept in mind that the method using the cold water irrigation alone is not adequate for screening out all abnormalities of caloric reaction and information can be derived from this test only when either a feeble response lasting for less than 90 seconds or lack of response is obtained. Otherwise the interpretation should be reserved until the hot water irrigation is applied.

The use of ENG has increased the sensitivity of vestibular examinations to the point that it is not always necessary to perform a complete caloric examination. All of the information revealed by the complete caloric examination can be obtained by the examination of spontaneous nystagmus and cold caloric tests. For example, if spontaneous nystagmus is not disclosed even with the eyes open in darkness and eyes closed, any significant difference in caloric reaction between right and left stimulation especially in the maximum slow phase speed may directly indicate a hypoexcitability of one side.

If spontaneous nystagmus toward either side is recorded on the ENG, the average slow phase speed of spontaneous nystagmus under the same visual condition as in the caloric test is considered to be the base line for evaluation the difference in the maximum slow phase speed of caloric nystagmus between both ears. Any significant difference thus obtained may indicate the presence of hypoexcitability on the side showing a lesser reaction or hyperexcitability of the other side (Fig. 46).

ii) Alternate cold and hot caloric test (FITZGERALD and HALLPIKE, 1942)

This method, different from the simple caloric test using cold stimulation alone, enables one to divide abnormal findings into a hypoexcitability and a directional preponderance by the application of cold and hot stimulations which are equidistant (7 °C) from body temperature.

Procedure (Fig. 47): The test is carried out with the patient lying supine on a couch with the head raised 30 degrees above the horizontal. The stimulus temperatures are 30 °C and 44 °C. The water is led to the ear through a rubber tube with a pressure head of about 2 ft. The nozzle used has an internal diameter of 4 mm (Fig. 47), the quantity of water between 400 and 600 ml being delivered during the stimulus time of 40 seconds. The patient's gaze should be fixed straight ahead upon a convenient mark on the ceiling.

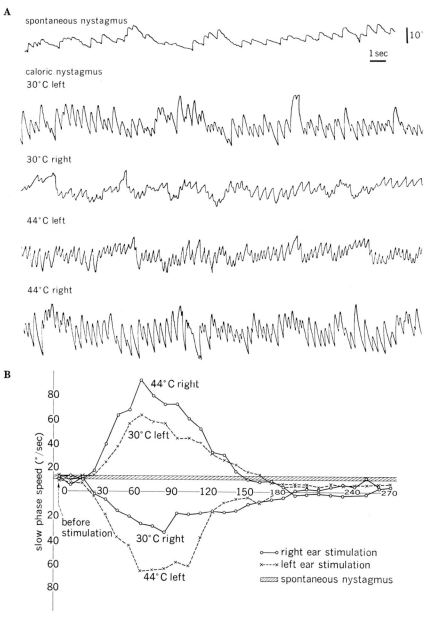

Fig. 46 Evaluation of the caloric test in a case with spontaneous nystagmus.
Usually in such cases the result of the alternate cold and hot caloric test is evaluated by using the maximum slow phase speed of caloric reaction. Each value in this case was 63°/sec in 30°C Left, 34 in 30°C Right, 66 in 44°C Left, and 92 in 44°C Right.
CP: (30°C Left+44°C Left)−(30°C Right+44°C Right)=(63+66)−(34+92)=3. DP: (30°C Left+44°C Right)+(30°C Right+44°C Left)=(63+92)−(34+66)=55. Therefore, this case was judged to have a DP to the right and no CP. However, this can be estimated from the intensity of the spontaneous nystagmus and the results of cold stimulation, even if the hot stimulation had not been performed. As shown in Fig. 46B, the real magnitude of the caloric reaction with 30°C stimulation to the left ear may be obtained by subtracting the average slow phase speed of spontaneous nystagmus (shaded bar−14°/sec) from the value of the induced nystagmus; 63−14=49, and that with 30°C to the right ear by adding the intensity of the spontaneous nystagmus to the value of induced nystagmus; 34+14=48. Since comparison between the values does not indicate any significant difference, the presence of CP can be denied.

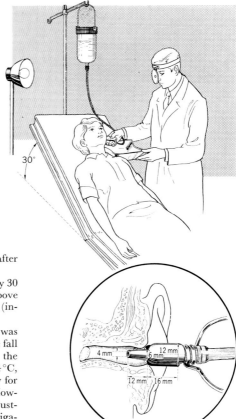

Fig. 47 Alternate cold and hot caloric test after
FITZGERALD and HALLPIKE (1942).
The patient lies supine with the head elevated by 30
degrees. The reservoir is placed about 2 feet above
the patient's external canal and the irrigator (in-
set) is introduced into the canal.
When the water of 44°C in the thermostat was
irrigated by using an ordinary rubber tube, the fall
in temperature in a room of 22°C between the
thermostat and the irrigation nozzle was 1.4°C,
although the water was allowed to follow freely for
more than one minute (HENRIKSSON, 1956). However, if the time between the completion of adjustment of water temperature and the start of irrigation is fixed, the temperature difference may be
constant and both ears can be stimulated equally.

Nystagmus is observed by using light reflected from a head mirror from a source above
and behind the patient's head, care being taken not to interrupt the patient's line of
fixation.

The time interval between the application of the stimulus and the end of the nystagmic
response is measured in seconds, the so-called latent period being thus neglected.

The tests are performed with an interval of at least five minutes in the following order;
30°C left ear, 30°C right ear, 44°C left ear, and 44°C right ear.   The results obtained
are recorded diagrammatically as shown in Fig. 48.

Interpretation: The duration of the cold responses is 120 seconds and of the hot responses
rather shorter, 100 seconds.   Interpretation is made from the mutual relationship of the four
responses, but not from the magnitude of each response.   Namely, the difference between
the left responses and the right responses, i.e., the left/right sensitivity difference: (30°C
Left + 44°C Left) − (30°C Right + 44°C Right), and directional preponderence, i.e.
the difference between reactions of 30°C Left and 44°C Right which consist of nystagmus
to the right, and reactions of 30°C Right and 44°C Left which consist of nystagmus to the
left: (30°C Left + 44°C Right) − (30°C Right + 44°C Left) are estimated in each
case.   When the magnitude of the difference is greater than 40 seconds, it is abnormal
(Table 2).   An abnormal Left/Right sensitivity difference is judged as canal paresis
(C. P.) of the side exhibiting a shorter duration.   If there is a directional preponderance,

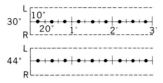

a. Normal

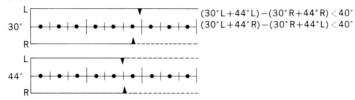

$(30°L+44°L)-(30°R+44°R)<40°$
$(30°L+44°R)-(30°R+44°L)<40°$

b. Right canal paresis (CP)

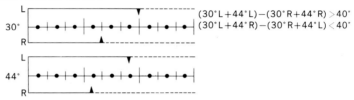

$(30°L+44°L)-(30°R+44°R)>40°$
$(30°L+44°R)-(30°R+44°L)<40°$

c. Directional preponderance to the left

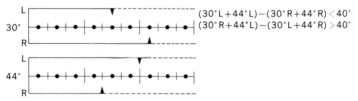

$(30°L+44°L)-(30°R+44°R)<40°$
$(30°R+44°L)-(30°L+44°R)>40°$

d. Combined type — Right CP+DP to the left

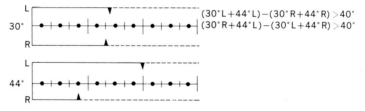

$(30°L+44°L)-(30°R+44°R)>40°$
$(30°R+44°L)-(30°L+44°R)>40°$

Fig. 48 Four types of calorigram.

The horizontal line represents time and three minutes are divided into intervals of 10 seconds. The duration of nystagmus is indicated by the solid line and the end point of nystagmus is indicated by the arrow head. Equations at the right of each calorigram express the results.

a) Normal: Difference in nystagmus duration between irrigation of both sides is less than 40 seconds. Difference between the reactions to the right and to the left is less than 40 seconds.

b) Right canal paresis (CP): Difference between nystagmus durations of right sided 30°C and 44°C stimulation and those of left sided 30°C and 44°C stimulation exceeds 40 seconds. Right sided reactions are shorter and the CP is named by the weaker side, i.e. right canal paresis.

c) Directional preponderance to the left: Difference between nystagmus durations to the left, i.e. (30°R+44°L) and those to the right, i.e. (30°L+44°R) is greater than 40 seconds. The DP is named to the stronger side, i.e. left directional preponderance.

d) Right CP plus DP to the left: The apparent difference between the right and left sides at 30°C from the right CP (See b) is canceled by the DP to left (See c), while the difference in the 44°C reactions is enhanced (Graphic addition of b+c=d).

Table 2 Normal values of nystagmus duration in the caloric test according to HALLPIKE. The duration of nystagmus was measured by direct observation (HALLPIKE et al., THOMSON, UEMURA et al.) or from the records obtained using PENG(Pfaltz) or ENG on eye opening in darkness (HENRIKSSON). The normal limit of each parameter can be estimated by the equation (mean $\pm$ 2×standard deviation) and it corresponds roughly to the rejection limit (5%). Thus, in the case of direct observation the abnormal value of CP or DP is more than 40 seconds.

	HALLPIKE et al. (1951)		THOMSEN (1953)		UEMURA et al. (1959)		PFALTZ (1957)		HENRIKSSON (1956)	
	Mean	St.Dev.	Mean	St.Dev.	Mean	St.Dev.	Mean	St.Dev.	Mean	St.Dev.
Total sensitivity $(30°L+30°R+44°L+44°R)$	420	60	425	50	420.3	45.2	515	125	618.9	82.3
The cold/hot sensitivity difference $(30°L+30°R)-(44°L+44°R)$	15.3	25.4	19.4	22.5	14.1	17.9	24.7	19.9	14.4	27.5
The left/right sensitivity difference $(30°L+44°L)-(30°R+44°R)$	−1.9	15.5	−0.5	11.6	−7.9	17.5	13.5	10.0	2.0	23.9
Directional preponderance $(30°L+44°R)-(30°R+44°L)$	−0.2	15.7	−3.7	17.3	1.5	18.0	30.6	26.1	−10.4	31.8

it is called D. P. to the side exhibiting a longer duration. Canal paresis and D. P. may occur in combination.

Canal paresis means paresis of the lateral semicircular canal. Since the difference between the left and right responses may be caused by the hypersensitivity of the other side, the condition that the reaction obtained by the cold or/and hot stimulation on that side is abnormally feeble should be required for interpretation of canal paresis. On the other hand, regarding the directional preponderance it is difficult to distinguish whether the nystagmus directed to one side is enhanced or the nystagmus directed to the other side is suppressed.

According to HALLPIKE (1955), D.P. to the lesion side occurs with lesions of the vestibular connection in the brain stem, of the vestibulocerebellar centers, and of the posterior part of one or other of the temporal lobes. D.P. to the intact side occurs in unilateral labyrinthine lesion probably due to a lesion of the utricle. Recently, however, some doubt has been raised as to the diagnostic significance of D.P. in signifying peripheral and central lesions (see below).

b. Discussion of the examination methods

The advantage of using the equidistant stimuli of 30 °C and 44 °C is that the results of the caloric test can be divided into the four types of normal, canal paresis (C. P.), D. P. and the combination of C. P. and D. P. However, several modifications have been reported, although the temperatures of water used for irrigation are generally 30 °C and 44 °C.

i) Amount of water and duration of irrigation

Originally the duration of irrigation was 40 seconds, thus the amount of water varied between 400 and 600 ml.

JONGKEES (1949, 1953) used an irrigation with 50 ml in order to obtain a reaction which was easily measured and to avoid great discomfort to the patient. ASCHAN et al. (1956) and STAHLE (1956, 1958) shortened the duration of irrigation to 30 seconds, sufficient time to cause a nystagmic reaction large enough to be recorded with ENG during eye closure,

Table 3 Values of the mean and standard deviation in various caloric test methods. HENRIKSSON and PFALTZ irrigated for 40 seconds and recorded nystagmus with ENG or PENG on eye opening in darkness; STAHLE irrigated for 30 seconds (approximately 100 ml) and used ENG on eye closure; OHTANI irrigated with 50 ml and used ENG on eye closure. Normal values can be estimated by the equation (mean $\pm 2 \times$ standard deviation).

	CP				DP			
	Duration (sec)		Maximum slow phase speed (°/sec)		Duration (sec)		Maximum slow phase speed (°/sec)	
	Mean	St. Dev.	Mean	St. Dev.	Mean	St. Dev.	Mean	St. Dev.
HENRIKSSON (1956)	2.0	23.9	−0.6	12.3	−10.4	31.8	0.5	10.5
PFALTZ (1957)	13.5	10.0	—	—	30.6	26.1	—	—
STAHLE (1956, 1958)	4	24	−1.0	5.2	−7	29	0.9	5.4
OHTANI (1962)	32.6	34.9	4.4	4.3	59.5	62.5	4.5	5.8

On the other hand, FRENZEL (1959) adopted a HALLPIKE's original method as a routine technique to be performed by a technician.

Because of the standard deviations of normal values which were obtained from various methods of irrigation (Table 3), it does not seem justified to shorten the duration of irrigation below 30 seconds or diminish the quantity of water below 100 ml.

ii)   Conditions for observation and recording

As DIX and HALLPIKE (1942) pointed out, direct observation of the induced nystagmus makes it easier to decide its end point. However, since the nystagmus induced by HALLPIKE's method is not always vigorous and its appearance is often influenced by the condition of illumination in the examination room, the use of Frenzel glasses should be recommended.

Application of ENG to record caloric nystagmus has been made popular as the equipment has improved and become easier to use. Recording is performed with the eyes closed or with the eyes open in darkness. The condition of closing the eyes, though used widely, often causes an irregularity of the nystagmic reaction, which results in the appearance of dysrhythmia even in normal subjects, and makes it difficult to analyse the entire reaction quantitatively. On the other hand, a marked suppression of the nystagmic reaction takes place when wearing Frenzel glasses or opening the eyes in light, as compared to the eyes closed condition or the eyes open in darkness condition. Consequently, recording caloric nystagmus with the eyes open in darkness is recommendable.

iii)   Evaluation

1) Judgement of the end point in nystagmic reaction.

JONGKEES (1953) introduced Arslan's method in which, on approaching the end point of the nystagmus, the examiner counts each nystagmic jerk and asks his assistant to record the intervals. When the interval exceeds 15 seconds for the first time, it is concluded that the previous jerk is the end point of the reaction. In addition to a decrease in nystagmus frequency and amplitude, the appearance of rapid eye movements toward other side (counterbeats) may be taken into consideration for judgement of the end point of caloric nystagmus (PFALTZ, 1957).

In general, the termination of caloric nystagmus seems to be less abrupt than that of the nystagmus induced by the rotation test, and there is a tendency to repeat such that the nystagmus pauses and reappears after its termination. Therefore, it is necessary to continue observation or recording for at least 10 seconds before judging that the nystagmus has ceased. We have adopted the 10 second interval for determining the end point of caloric nystagmus recorded with ENG.

2) Absolute vs. relative values (%).

A difference of e.g. 40 seconds between the left and right ears at an excitability level of 50 seconds per irrigation may be pathological, whereas the same difference of 40 seconds at a level of 300 seconds will fall within the normal limits. Thus the difference in excitability between the left and right ears or between the left and right directions was expressed in the percentage of the total excitability as follows (JONGKEES et al., 1962):

$$\text{C.P. } (\%) = \frac{(30°\text{L} + 44°\text{L}) - (30°\text{R} + 44°\text{R})}{30°\text{L} + 30°\text{R} + 44°\text{L} + 44°\text{R}} \times 100$$

$$\text{D.P. } (\%) = \frac{(30°\text{L} + 44°\text{R}) - (30°\text{R} + 44°\text{L})}{30°\text{L} + 30°\text{R} + 44°\text{L} + 44°\text{R}} \times 100$$

However, when results of testing the same 293 patients were interpreted by means of the absolute and relative values as to canal paresis and D.P., no significant difference in the positive rate of pathological findings were found.

3) Interpretation by using the parameters other than duration of nystagmus
Application of ENG or PENG made it possible to perform accurate measurement of amplitude, frequency and eye speed of the slow phase of the nystagmic reaction, in addition to the duration of nystagmus. Among these parameters of nystagmus, the maximum eye speed of the slow phase was regarded from experimental evidence to be the most sensitive parameter of the intensity of stimulus used. Nystagmus duration increases rapidly as the differential of the temperature of water used for irrigation and body temperature from 0 to $\pm 7°$C, however a differential greater than $\pm 7°$C only causes slight increment in nystagmus duration (JONGKEES, 1949).

HENRIKSSON (1955) devised a method for direct measurement of the eye speed in the slow phase of nystagmus and suggested the possibility of detecting abnormal findings from the eye speed of the slow phase, which could not be deduced from the nystagmus duration. KOCH et al. (1959) disclosed in clinical cases a higher percentage of D.P. and canal paresis when judged by the nystagmus duration rather than by the maximum eye speed of slow phase, however they attempted to explain their results concerning canal paresis by the inadequateness of the nystagmus duration for judging the reactivity of the peripheral organ. We, however, could not find any significant difference in the positive rate between both methods of judgment on 293 patients.

c. **Significance of the caloric test in topical diagnosis**
Although a hypoexcitability of the tested ear to caloric stimulation (canal paresis) may be caused by lesions present in the peripheral labyrinth or in the vestibular nerve, the diagnostic evaluation of the phenomena described below has been a subject of dispute.

i) *Directional preponderance (D. P.)*
Attention has been drawn to the directional preponderance of induced labyrinthine nystagmus, since FITZGERALD and HALLPIKE (1942) revealed D.P. of caloric nystagmus to the side of the lesion in all of 10 cases with a lesion of one temporal lobe. Furthermore, they confined the lesion responsible for this abnormality to the posterior part of the temporal lobe (CARMICHAEL et al., 1954, 1955).

The occurrence of D.P. in unilateral cerebral lesions was variously reported to be 89% (48 out of 54 cases) (ANDERSEN et al., 1954), 38% (38 out of 101 cases) (ANDERSEN, 1954), and 43% (29 out of 68 cases) (KIRSTEIN and PREBER, 1954). Although SANDBERG and ZILSTORFF-PEDERSEN (1961) found D.P. in 60% (21) out of 35 patients with diseases affecting mainly the temporal lobe, 6 cases, contrary to the results of CARMICHAEL et al. (1954, 1955), had involvement of only the anterior part of the temporal lobe. Moreover, RIESCO-MACCLURE (1964) found D.P. in 28% (26) out of 94 cases with brain lesions of different nature and localization, in which the lesions were not limited to the temporal lobe.

On the other hand, HAKAS and KORNHUBER (1959) examined 201 cases with localized cerebral lesions by means of the rotation test with the eyes closed and found D.P. in 31%. The directions of D.P. seen in these cases were more likely to be toward the unaffected side, and also their lesions were not exclusively confined to the temporal lobe. HOFMANN (1962) could not find D.P. in any of 5 patients with cerebral tumor by means of the rotation test, and KOIKE et al. (1967) found D.P. of caloric nystagmus to the affected side in only 3 out of 15 cases with tumors of the temporal lobe during eye closure.

CARMICHAEL et al. (1961) explained the discrepancy in the results by the findings that D.P. of induced nystagmus to the side of the lesion occurred because of the maintenance of optic fixation in direct forward gaze and was abolished or reversed under the condition of eye closure or eye opening in darkness. By examining 34 cases with lesions of one cerebral hemisphere under both conditions of visual fixation and eye closure, however, BADER and KORNHUBER (1965) denied the significance of D.P. of caloric nystagmus for topographic diagnosis of cortical lesions of the temporal lobe.

In conclusion, evaluation of the data published to date indicates that no information concerning topical diagnosis is revealed from the presence or absence of D.P. in caloric testing.

ii)   Dysrhythmia

Disordered rhythm in the appearance of caloric nystagmus has become clearly demonstrable with the application of ENG. As shown in Fig. 49B, caloric nystagmus may disappear repeatedly for 5 to 10 seconds during the duration of the caloric reaction.

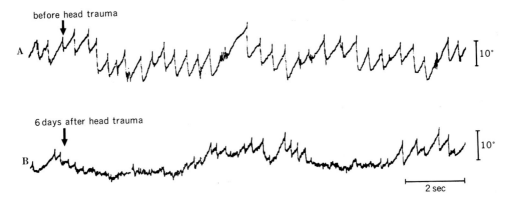

Fig. 49   Dysrhythmia—ENG records of caloric nystagmus with the eyes open in darkness before and after head trauma.
At the time record A was taken, caloric nystagmus appeared normal. Record B was taken six days after head trauma. Prominent dysrhythmia is noted. The arrows indicate 80 seconds after the irrigation of 5 ml water at 20°C to the right ear.

Dysrhythmia was postulated by ASCHAN et al. (1956) to be related to disturbed cerebral function. RIESCO-MACCLURE and STROUD (1960) and RIESCO-MACCLURE (1964) also reported that dysrhythmia appeared particularly with lesions of the midline structures probably due to lack of cerebellar influence over the vestibular nuclei. In this case, the dysrhythmia was differentiated from that seen in the normal subjects by asking the subject to fix his eyes on an object. MEHRA (1964), however, observed this phenomenon of dysrhythmia in some of normal subjects even though the subject was asked to fixate.

From our experience, dysrhythmia is frequently found in fresh cases of head trauma during eye opening in darkness. The dysrhythmia of caloric nystagmus during eye closure, however, cannot

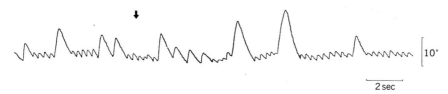

Fig. 50   Another type of dysrhythmia seen in a case with cerebellar tumor.
The record was taken with the eyes open in darkness after the irrigation of 5 ml water at 20°C to the left ear. The arrow indicates 50 seconds after the beginning of irrigation.

be regard as abnormal, since it often appears in normal subjects when they are tired or sleepy. Thus it may be postulated that a lack of aletrness is responsible for dysrhythmia.

Another type of dysrhythmia was found in a case with cerebellar tumor (Fig. 50). An impairment of the rhythm concerning the genesis of the quick and slow phases without concomitant change in eye speed may cause an irregularity in the amplitude and frequency of nystagmus.

iii) Perverted nystagmus

When the nystagmus induced by caloric stimulation to the lateral semicircular canal is vertical or oblique, it is designated as perverted nystagmus.

RIESCO-MACCLURE (1964) found perverted nystagmus in 8 out of 95 cases of intracranial lesions, and thought that it is a clinical expression of a partial destructive lesion of the vestibular area on the floor of the fourth ventricle. UEMURA and COHEN (1972, 1973) were able to produce perverted nystagmus in rhesus monkeys with a discrete electrolytic lesion in the rostral medial vestibular nucleus. The hot stimulation to the unaffected side caused downward nystagmus and the cold stimulation caused upward diagonal nystagmus. This was attributed to some disturbance of the commissural fibers between the vestibular nuclei of the both sides.

iv) Loss of the quick phase of caloric nystagmus

Although it has been realized for a long time that brainstem lesions may produce loss of the quick phase of induced nystagmus, little information as to precise location of lesions responsible for this abnormality could be obtained from clinical cases. However, loss of the quick phase has been produced experimentally in monkeys (SHANZER and BENDER, 1959; BENDER and SHANZER, 1964; COHEN et al., 1968). Localized lesion of the paramedian zone of the pontine reticular formation appears to result in loss of the quick phase of induced nystagmus to the ipsilateral side and ipsilateral paresis of conjugate gaze.

On the other hand, during the course of recovery following unilateral lesions of the medial longitudinal fasciculus, monocular recording of ENG may reveal diminished eye speed in the quick phase of caloric nystagmus as well as in the saccades only in the ipsilateral adductive eye (COHEN, 1971).

v) Vestibular recruitment

It is of special interest whether the vestibular system has a phenomenon similar to auditory recruitment which is useful for differentiating cochlear and retrocochlear lesions. Several attempts had been made by caloric testing to study the presence of vestibular recruitment (AZZI et al., 1953; OKAMOTO, 1959; IKEDA, 1964). Recently LITTON and McCABE (1966) have demonstrated in patients with Ménière's disease that, although the caloric reaction was consistently weaker in the involved than in the normal ear, the caloric reaction of the diseased labyrinth increased as the stimulus intensity was increased. Moreover, STEFFEN et al. (1970) made it possible to examine a relationship between the stimulus intensity and the reaction magnitude by continuously changing temperatures of the irrigation solution. In these cases the parameter of nystagmus used was the maximum speed of the slow phase.

TOROK (1970) applied weak and strong caloric stimulations to normal and abnormal cases and the ratio of the frequency counts to both stimuli is estimated at the culmination. When strong stimulation elicited a disproportionate increase or decrease in comparison to weak stimulation, it was termed a recruitment or decruitment. Recruitment was found in labyrinthine disease and decruitment was found in a variety of central nervous system pathology.

Experimental evidence was obtained from monkeys with lesions of the nerve trunk of the vestibular nerve, in which the maximum eye speed of slow phase increased very little or not at all with increasing strength of caloric stimulation (UEMURA and COHEN, 1972, 1973).

vi) Other abnormalities of caloric reaction

There are some other abnormalities such as distortion of the culmination phenomenon (TOROK, 1957; GULICK and PFALTZ, 1964), cochleovestibular dissociation (RIESCO-MACCLURE, 1964), vestibular hyperexcitability without concomitant autonomic irritation or sensation (SUZUKI, 1961) and appearance of the second phase of caloric nystagmus (MORIMOTO et al., 1963). However, their isolated appearance may not provide clear evidence for topographic localization of the dysfunction.

The caloric test has been long regarded as an essential part of the routine vestibular evaluation and the advantage that alternate cold and hot caloric stimulation is able to distinguish clearly between a directional preponderance of induced nystagmus and a hypoexcitability of the labyrinth has been emphasized. Although doubt was cast on the topical evaluation of D.P., the D.P. may be interpreted as a sensitive sign of vestibular tonus difference between the both sides.   As recording of ENG with the eyes closed and open in darkness has raised the detection rate of spontaneous and provoked nystagmus, it seems likely that the discovery of a D.P. solely by means of the caloric test has become obsolete.

Recently, JONGKEES and PHILIPSZOON(1964) stated an extreme view that there are only few cases in which the caloric test will give new information after the posture test and the audiometry has been performed.   However, the audiogram evaluates only the cochlear portion of the labyrinth, and the presence of spontaneous or provoked nystagmus does not always indicate the involved side.   The caloric test, if abnormal, may provide clear evidence of the side of the dysfunction, i.e. canal paresis is caused exclusively by peripheral labyrinthine or VIIIth nerve damage.

In conclusion, if ENG is available and some abnormality is revealed by recording, structural or functional damage of the vestibular system may be verified.   However, if clear documentation of the side and grade of the damage is needed, the caloric test is indispensable.

2.   The Rotation Test

a.   Vestibular responses elicited by rotary stimulation

i)   Evaluation of semicircular canal function

Since angular acceleration is the normal mode of stimulation of the semicircular canals, it may be expected that investigating the effects of this stimulus can yield valuable information about canal function.   To produce angular acceleration the subjects should be rotated at increasing or decreasing speeds.   If responses of the horizontal canal are to be tested, the seated subject should have his head tilted 30 degrees forward, as this brings the plane of the horizontal canal into the plane of rotation.   Thus, the effects of angular acceleration will act primarily on this canal.   The effective stimuli are positive angular acceleration at the onset of turning and negative forces at the moment of stopping.   This angular acceleration induces cupular deviation consequent upon the endolymph flow (MACH-BREUER).   The degree of cupular deviation is proportional to the magnitude of acceleration or deceleration and has been shown to modify the ongoing activity in the VIIIth nerve.   This process is generally thought to be involved in the generation of nystagmus.   Thus, when a subject is rotated with the head tilted forward by 30 degrees a horizontal nystagmus is elicited to the same side as the turning.   This is called a perrotatory nystagmus.   When the turning is stopped, horizontal nystagmus will also be evoked but will be directed to the opposite side.   This is called a postrotatory nystagmus.

The purpose of rotation tests is to observe the quantitative relation between the acceleratory (or deceleratory) stimuli and the labyrinthine reaction as indicated by nystagmus. It is convenient that not only the parameters of nystagmus but also the stimuli parameters, i.e. the magnitude of angular acceleration can be expressed numerically.   This is one advantage of the rotation test, however one drawback is that the evaluation of unilateral labyrinthine function by this test is difficult, as both labyrinths are simultaneously stimulated by rotation of the head.   According to EDWALD's law, the labyrinth of the same side as the direction of turning is responsible for eliciting perrotatory nystagmus, while postrotatory nystagmus is elicited chiefly by excitation of the opposite labyrinth.   Some investigators believe that EDWALD's law is completely invalid while others find it true in part. To test the effects of angular acceleration on the bilateral horizontal canals the following three experiments were designed.

ii) Experimental investigation of the effects of rotation.

(1)   The pressure changes in the lateral semicircular canals of pigeons were investigated by a strain gauge manometer during angular deceleration.   Figure 51 illustrates the record of intracanalicular pressure taken from a single canal during rotation in both directions.

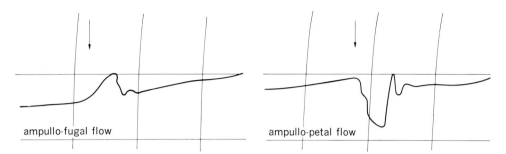

ampullo-fugal flow   ampullo-petal flow

Fig. 51   Pressure change in the pigeon's lateral semicircular canal recorded during angular deccelera-
tion.
A Pito's tube was inserted in the lateral semicircular canal.   The intracanal pressure was transmitted to
a straingauge manometer and was recorded on a pen-writer.   When rotation of 30 degrees per second
was suddenly stopped pressure chage in the canal subject to ampullopetal forces were greater than those
of the one subject to ampullofugal forces.

Changes in pressure were most marked when sudden stopping of rotation produced ampullopetal cupular deviation.   This larger pressure change should correspond to more marked
cupular deviation with forces in the ampullopetal direction than with those in the ampullofugal direction.

(2)   Deviation of the cupula of the horizontal canal in response to rotation was examined morphologically.   A pigeon was subjected to rotation and its head was rapidly
frozen at the moment of cessation of rotation.   Thus the morphological deviation of
the cupula could be preserved for later histological investigation.   The pigeon's head
was immersed in liquid nitrogen, and was fixed for several weeks in 1.0% mercury chloride
in ethanol.   Upon dissection of the horizontal canals, as shown in Fig. 52, the right
cupula, subject to ampullopetal forces, appeared to be deviated more strongly than its
fellow of the opposite side.

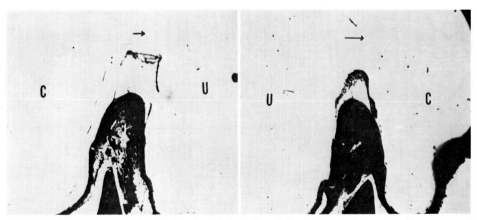

Fig. 52   The cupular deflexion in the pigeon's lateral semicircular canal observed at the moment of
cessation of rotation.
Note that the utriculo-petal deviation of the cupula predominated over the utriculo-fugal deviation
of the opposite side.   U indicates the utricular side.   Arrow points in the direction of endolymph flow.

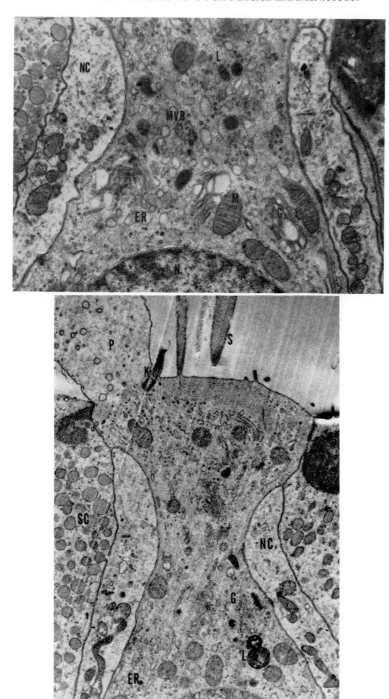

Fig. 53 The effects of rotatory stimulation on the sensory epithelium of the crista ampullaris.
Upper picture shows the supranuclear part of a type-I cell in the lateral ampulla stimulated by ampullopetal flow: Most of the mitochondria (M) were not altered morphologically. The endoplasmic reticulum (ER) showed some swelling. Golgi vacuoles (G) were dilated. Lysosome-like bodies (L) and multivesicular bodies (MVB) are seen.   ×18000.
Lower picture shows supranuclear part of a type-I cell in the lateral ampulla stimulated by ampullofugal flow: No dilatation of either endoplasmic reticulum (ER) or Golgi complex (G) were observed but several dense bodies (L) are noted.   ×14000.

(3)   The sensory epithelium was examined after rotation.   Guinea pigs were subjected to repeated angular deceleration in one direction for a period of 24 hours.   The labyrinths were then removed and the sensory epithelium was subjected to histological examination including electron microscopy.   As explained in the legend of Fig. 53, morphological changes were more pronounced on the side subjected to ampullopetal forces.

Thus, although the effects of angular acceleration were demonstrated bilaterally and therefore EWALD's law does not seem to be strictly true, it may be stated that there is a unilateral predominance of the effects of rotary stimuli.

From the clinical point of view, this theory is still the most satisfactory of all hypotheses and it provides a convenient explanation for the results of rotation tests which seems to fit the clinical data.

b.   Types of rotation tests

Rotation tests may be divided into those which test perrotatory nystagmus and those which test postrotatory nystagmus.   A representative list of the various methods is presented in Table 4.   In particular, the test of perrotatory nystagmus by *self-recording cupulometry* and that of postrotatory nystagmus by *manual cupulometry* will be described.

Table 4   Kinds of rotation test.

Method	Mode of rotation	Parameter
BÁRÁNY's method	Forced-turning (20 sec; 10 revolution)	Postrotatory nystagmus (inspection method)
GRAHE's method	Short-turning (1/4 or 1/2 revolution)	Perrotatory nystagmus (palpation method)
Cupulometry (EGMOND, JONGKEES)	Subliminal rotation and stop	Postrotatory nystagmus and sensation
A-D test (HALLPIKE, HOOD)	Acceleration and deceleration ($4°/sec^2$)	Perrotatory nystagmus (ENG)
Deceleration test (KOBRAK, WUST)	Gradual decrease of rotation (5 or 6 revolution)	Per- and postrotatory nystagmus (ENG)
Liminal rotation test (MONTAGNDON)	Acceleration and deceleration (1, 3, $5°/sec^2$)	Perrotatory nystagmus (ENG)
Pendular rotation test (BÉKÉSY, GREINER, MATSUNAGA, SETOGUCHI)	Pendular rotation	Perrotatory nystagmus and sensation (ENG)
Superliminal rotation test (TOKUMASU)	Superliminal rotation and stop	Per- and postrotatory nystagmus (ENG)
Self-recording cupulometry (HOZAWA, SASAKI)	Acceleration and deceleration (2, 6, $10°/sec^2$)	Latency time of perrotatory nystagmus (television)

c.   Self-recording cupulometry

The patient sits in an electrically driven turning chair with the head bent forward at 30 degrees.   Eye movements are observed by a television camera placed in front of the subject's eyes and secured so as to rotate with the chair (Fig.54).   The onset of nystagmus can be precisely determined by viewing the eyes in this way.

Fig. 55 is the record of the velocity of an electrically driven rotating chair.   If a subject is seated in this chair and (Step 1), constant angular acceleration is applied (A–B), a perrotatory nystagmus may be induced.

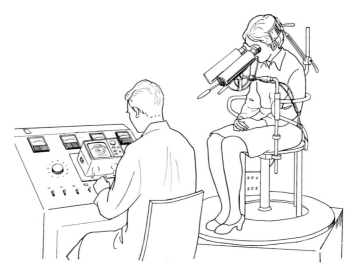

Fig. 54 The testing method of self-recording cupulometry.
The patient sits in the electrically driven turning chair with the head bent forward at 30 degrees.
During the test the eye movement is observed through a television camera in front of the eyes.
The examiner rotates the chair in the manner previously described. During the test, the speed
of the chair is recorded on a penoscillograph.

However, as noted there is some time lag between the onset of rotation at A and the
onset of nystagmus at B.   This delay or latency is called La.   If the acceleration of the
chair is switched off, to the constant velocity rotation as soon as nystagmus appears, i.e.
at B, then the distance along the base line or time axis from A to B is the latency to onset
of nystagmus or La. (Step 2), constant velocity rotation is then continued until nystagmus
stops.   (Step 3), then constant deceleration is applied at C and switched off at D as soon
as nystagmus in the opposite direction appears.   Ld in Fig. 55a is, by analogy, the latency to onset of nystagmus during deceleration.   If La equals Ld then A and D will
be at equal height from the base line.   If Ld is shorter, then D will be higher than A as
in Fig. 55a.

According to EWALD (1892), if clockwise acceleration is applied, the right labyrinth will be
primarily active while during deceleration the left labyrinth will be mainly responsible for evoked
nystagmus.

Using this procedure the sensitivity of the labyrinths to acceleration and deceleration can
thus be automatically recorded by referring to the penwriter record of the velocity of the
rotating chair.   Therefore we have named this test the self-recording cupulometry.

Any difference between La and Ld will become more easily visible if the test is
repeated three times in succession.   Thus, if there is a difference between the responses of
the two labyrinths the thrice performed self-recording cupulogram shows an increasing
divergence from the base line (Fig. 55b).   This is called the divergence phenomenon.
This rotation test is performed mainly to detect the presence or absence of this divergence
phenomenon.

i)   *The testing method*

The principles of the effects of stimulation were previously delineated.   We now propose
to use stimuli of ± 2, 6, and 10 deg/sec^2. (Acceleratory or deceleratory stimuli of 2 deg/
sec are relatively weak while those of 10 deg/sec^2 are relatively strong.)   As stated, during
the application of these rotations the velocity of the chair is recorded with a pen writer
thus generating the self-recording cupulogram.

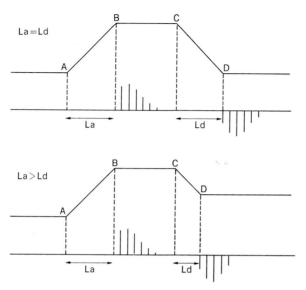

Fig. 55 a   Self-recording cupulometry recording of the velocity of the rotating chair.

A:	Beginning of acceleration	AB:	Constant angular acceleration
B:	Terminating of acceleration	BC:	Rotation with constant velocity
	(=onset of perrotatory ny.)	CD:	Deceleration with the same magni-
C:	Beginning of deceleration		tude as acceleration
D:	Terminating of deceleration	La:	Latency time, acceleration
	(=onset of perrotatory ny.)	Ld:	Latency time, deceleration

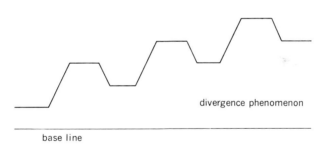

Fig. 55 b   The divergence phenomenon observed in self-recording cupulometry.
If there is a difference of sensitivity between right and left labyrinth as in Fig. 55a, the self-recording cupulogram, when repeated 3 times, shows an increasing divergence from the base line.   Self-recording cupulometry is a test to detect the presence or absence of this divergence phenomenon.

ii)   Classification of self-recording cupulograms

The self-recording cupulogram may be classified into three types (Fig. 56).

Type I: The normal type in which the divergence phenomenon is not observed, and the final point is always on the base line.

Type II: The divergence type in which the divergence phenomenon is observed at all three stimuli.

Type III: The reversion type in which the self-recording cupulogram shows a divergence with an acceleration of 2 or 6 deg/sec^2, but reverts to the base line with an increase of acceleration.

iii)   Diagnostic value

In this test, 85% of the 156 cases with vertigo were found to be of Type II or Type III

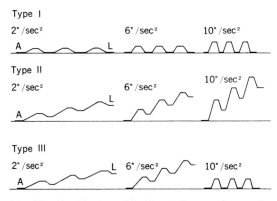

Fig. 56 Classification of "self-recording cupulogram."
Type I (normal type): The effect of acceleration and deceleration are identical. The final point (L) is always on the base line.
Type II (divergence type): The self-recording cupulogram always show a divergence from the base line. This type is caused by a "directional preponderance". Type III (reversion type): The self-recording cupulogram showing divergence with a weaker stimulation ($2°/\text{sec}^2$) reverts to the base line in accordance with the increase of stimulation ($10°/\text{sec}^2$). This type is found exclusively in cases of peripheral lesion, but not of central lesions.

i.e. divergence or reversion. Moreover, the reversion type was found exclusively in cases of peripheral vestibular lesion (Table 5).

If the reversion phenomenon appears the pathologic side may be indicated. Thus from Fig. 56 Type III it may be deduced that the right side is defective as the latency in response to weak stimulation of 2 and 6 deg/sec² was longer with acceleration than with deceleration, however in response to strong stimulation of 10 deg/sec² the latency was equal in both directions, i.e. reversion phenomenon.

An example, in a case of Ménière's disease, is illustrated in Fig. 57. The patient showed the reversion type of cupulogram. The self-recording cupulogram taken from a case of brainstem tumor showed divergence, but no reversion (Fig. 58). In Fig. 59, the reversion phenomenon is similar in appearance to auditory recruitment and was therefore thought to be a sign peculiar to peripheral vestibular disease.

iv) Experimental investigation of the reversion phenomenon

It was attempted to clarify the origin of the reversion phenomenon by the following basic experiments. First, a cat was prepared with a large unilateral vestibular nuclear

Table 5 Results of self-recording cupulometry.

Case	Type I	Type II	Type III	Total
Peripheral lesion				
Ménière's disease	1	0	24	25
Other disease	6	0	26	32
Acoustic tumor	0	6	1	7
Central lesion				
Cerebellum, brainstem	1	16	0	17
Others	4	19	0	23
Total	12	41	51	104

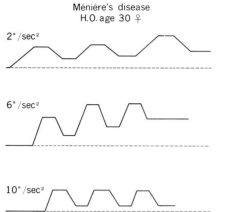

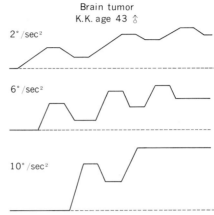

Fig. 57 Self-recording cupulogram observed in a case of Ménière's disease. The reversion type is demonstrated.

Fig. 58 Self-recording cupulogram observed in a case of brain tumor. The divergence type is demonstrated.

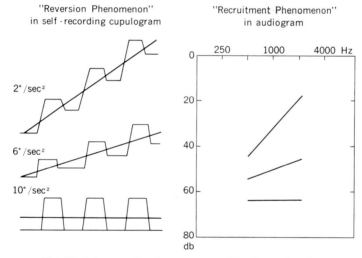

Fig. 59 The reversion phenomenon and its diagnostic value.
This phenomenon is similar in appearance to auditory recruitment, and was thought to be a sign peculiar to a peripheral vestibular lesion.

lesion produced by a stereotaxically implanted electrode and subsequently verified histologically. This cat showed divergence but no reversion. Next, in a second cat, the effect of compressing the vestibular nerve by stuffing bone wax into the internal auditory canal was observed. The cat showed divergence but no reversion. In third and fourth cats saccular or utricular nerve lesion were produced by otomicrosurgery. These cats also displayed no reversion. Finally, the influence of streptomycin sulfate on the labyrinth was observed. Streptomycin solution was injected into a guinea pig's tympanic cavity, and polarizing currents were applied to facilitate entry into the labyrinth. The reversion phenomena (Fig. 60a) was induced in this animal. The pathologic changes in Type I and Type II cells of the crista ampullaris were then studied with electron microscopy. It was noted that the pathological changes were most marked in Type I rather than in Type II cells (Fig. 60b).

From the results of these experiments, it was confirmed that the reversion phenomenon could be induced in cases of end organ injury. Judging from the difference of vulnerability between Type I and Type II cells in the crista ampullaris, the reversion phenomenon may be related more strongly to damage of Type I rather than Type II hair cells.

v) In summary, the advantages of this test procedure are (a) the time required to complete this test is about 15 minutes, (b) during the test the patient does not feel any discomfort, and (c) the response decline phenomenon i.e. adaptation, such as observed in other rotation tests, does not appear. We propose that self-recording cupulometry may be useful in order to differentiate between peripheral vestibular and central lesions.

d. Manual cupulometry

In order to study the cupulo-endolymphatic mechansim of the semicircular canals in a quantitative manner, EGMOND and JONGKEES (1948) introduced their method of cupulometry. This method uses one pure stimulus, deceleration, after elimination of all other interfering factors. The duration of the postrotatory nystagmus and sensation are measured and graphically recorded (cupulogram): the abscissa expresses the magnitude of stimulation on a logarithmic scale in deg/sec, the ordinate expresses the duration of postrotatory nystagmus and sensation in seconds.

Since the duration of response is proportional to the logarithm of the stimulus intensity, the normal cupulogram describes a straight line or course. Analysis of the cupulogram is useful in evaluating labyrinthine function. However, the cupulometry has the disadvantage that to eliminate the interfering stimulus of acceleration, the patient must be turned with a constant subliminal acceleration long enough to make sure that all reactions have subsided. This "long-turning method" often causes tiredness in the patient and the subsequent lack of maintenance of arousal, which may influence the results of the test. In order to maintain the advantages of cupulometry, while eliminating the above-mentioned shortcomings, another method of manual cupulometry has been developed.

i)   The method of manual cupulometry

A quiet dimly room is best for this test. The patient sits in the manually rotated chair with his head inclined so that the plane of rotation conforms with that of the lateral semicircular canals. After placing Frenzel glasses on the patient, he is instructed to close his eyes. The examiner then grasps the chair and walks gradually around increasing the length of his step until he reaches the requried speed of rotation. It is important for the examiner to walk softly so that the patient is not distracted. It is convenient to attach a tachometer to the chair so that the examiner can have some measure of the velocity of the chair (Fig. 61). After three revolutions at the required speed, the examiner stops the chair suddenly and instructs the patient to open his eyes so that nystagmus can be observed. The examiner can accurately perform this turning method with only a little practice. Accurate subliminal acceleration is not essential, but one should try to accelerate as slowly as possible and to maintain constant speed during the last three revolutions. Turning can be stopped at speeds of 20, 30 and 60 degrees per second. Thus measurements should be carried out a total of six times (3 clockwise and 3 counterclockwise rotations). In order that no influence remain from the previous turning it is necessary to rest for two minutes between measurements. Including the turning, observation of nystagmus and the rest period, this test can be performed in about fifteen minutes. This is about 1/3 of the time required for the original method of cupulometry.

ii)   The parameters of the test

The cupulogram of the original method consists of four lines, two for nystagmus and two for sensation, but postrotatory sensation is much too unreliable to be routinely used.

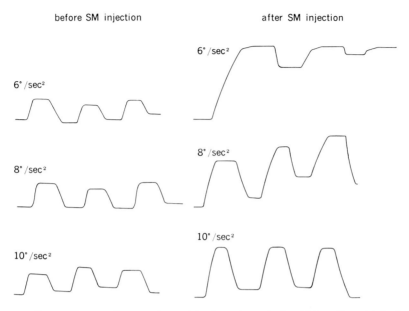

before SM injection

after SM injection

6°/sec²

6°/sec²

8°/sec²

8°/sec²

10°/sec²

10°/sec²

Fig. 60 a Self-recording cupulogram observed in the guinea pig in which unilateral labyrinth was affected by streptomycin.

The guinea pig showed the reversion type after being treated with streptomycin.   Pathological changes were observed in Type I and Type II cells of the crista ampullaris by electron microscopy.   It was noted that the pathological changes were more marked in Type I than in Type II cells (Fig. 60b).

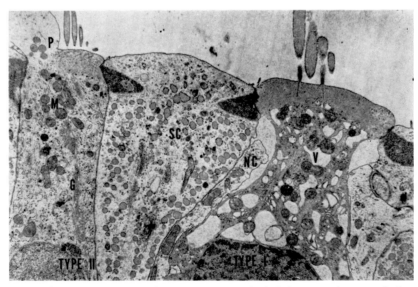

Fig. 60 b In the supernuclear part of a Type I cell pathological changes such as vacuole-formation, abnormal pigmentation and mitochondrial degeneration can be observed.   In a Type II cell such remarkable changes are not observed.

NC:	Nerve chalice	G:	Golgi complex
V:	Vacuole	SC:	Supporting cell
M:	Mitochondria		

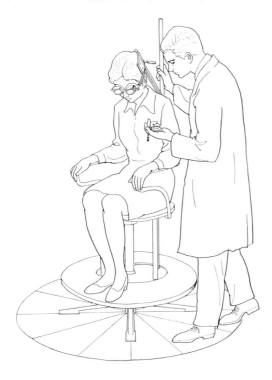

Fig. 61 The instruments used for manual cupulometry.

Therefore, the sensation cupulogram has been neglected. On the other hand, nystagmus duration was found to be more reliable than other parameters such as jerk-number, frequency, amplitude or eye-speed. Nystagmus duration can be measured simply with a stop watch. For clinical purposes, measurement of this parameter can be adequately performed by inspection under Frenzel glasses. The onset and termination of postrotatory nystagmus are so evident that even a relatively untrained examiner can catch them. (It

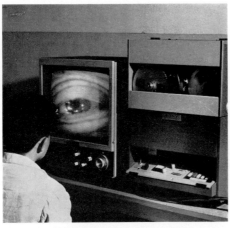
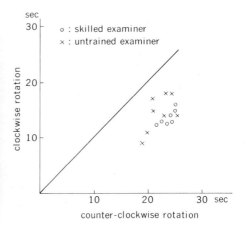

Fig. 62 Variation of nystagmus duration measured by inspection method.
By observing TV videotape in which postrotatory nystagmus was previously recorded, the examiner measured nystagmus duration. Difference of measured value between skilled and untrained examiners was very little. In this graph abscissa shows nystagmus duration after clockwise rotation and ordinate shows that of counter-clockwise rotation.

has been observed that there was very little difference in the results of skilled and untrained examiners when they measured the duration of nystagmus recorded on TV videotape.) (Fig. 62).

Thus, nystagmus duration is measured and plotted graphically in the same manner as in the original method of cupulometry. On the abscissa the magnitude of stimulation is expressed on a logarithmic scale in degrees per second, and on the ordinate the nystagmus duration is expressed in seconds. This is called the nystagmus cupulogram.

iii) *Classification of nystagmus cupulograms*

Normal cupulogram: The graph lines take a straight course. The cupulogram of clockwise rotation is identical with that of counterclockwise rotation (Fig. 63). The difference in nystagmus duration between clockwise and counter-clockwise rotation lies within five seconds.

Pathological cupulogram: These may be classified into two types, namely, the parellel type and the crossing type (Fig. 64).

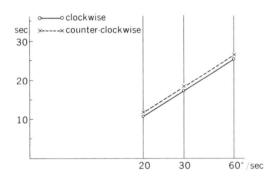

Fig. 63 Normal cupulogram.
Abscissa: velocity of rotation, ordinate: duration of nystagmus.

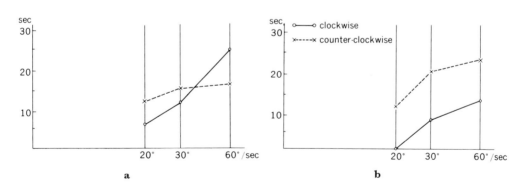

Fig. 64 Pathological cupulogram.
a: Crossing type,   b: Parallel type.   Further explanation is in the text.

iv) *Accuracy of manual cupulometry*

In order to test the accuracy of this method, a revolving room was devised as shown in Fig. 65.

This room may be rotated electrically with constant angular acceleration $(0.13-0.77$ deg/sec$^2)$ at speeds from 12 deg/sec to 120 deg/sec. By using this room, extravestibular influences are excluded and the original cupulometry may be performed very precisely.

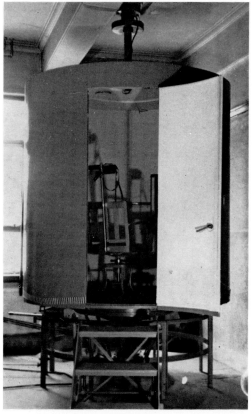

Fig. 65 Revolving room for testing labyrinthine reactions.
When the door is closed, extralabyrinthine
stimuli are excluded. Rotation from speeds of
12°/sec to 60°/sec are possible.

When the difference was evaluated between manual cupulometry and original cupulometry, a correlation was observed as shown in Fig. 66. The response type for the same
patient by manual cupulometry was identical with the results of the original cupulometry
as shown in Fig. 67.

From the above mentioned results, it may be seen that manual cupulometry is a simple
and reliable method to be used as a "routine test".

v)   Clinical value of this test

Value as a routine test: As this test can be carried out with a manually rotated chair,
requiring only fifteen minutes per patient, it is suitable as a routine test.

Diagnostic value: A pathological cupulogram was observed in 75% of 150 cases with
vertigo.   There were crossing type cupulograms observed in 38% of the cases with peripheral vestibular disturbances.   In this type, the steeper line indicated the diseased side.
This phenomenon seemed to be caused by "vestibular recruitment".   When Hallpike's
caloric test was carried out, "canal paresis" was often observed.   On the other hand, with
the parallel type cupulogram, central or peripheral vestibular disturbances are indicated
and, when Hallpike's caloric test was carried out, "directional preponderance" was often
observed.

Value for evaluating the effect of treatment: Changes in the cupulogram during treatment
of 160 cases of aural vertigo were observed.   In the parallel type cupulogram the width
between the two lines decreased in accordance with the improvement of vertigo, and
increased with the exacerbation of symptoms.   From these results it was shown that the
effectiveness of treatment for aural vertigo could be evaluated by this test.

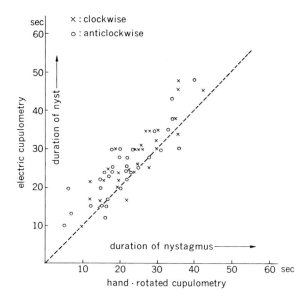

Fig. 66 Comparison of duration of nystagmus in the two methods of cupulometry.
The graph shows a high degree of correlation between duration of nystagmus measured by electric and hand cupulometry.

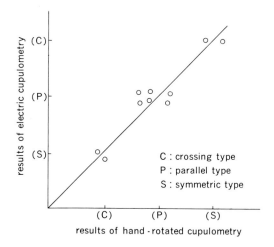

Fig. 67 Comparison of diagnosis in the two methods of cupulometry.

Manual cupulometry is also a useful method for evaluating the prognosis of vertigo.   Two
questions which arise in relation to vertigo are: 1) "Is the present treatment effective?" and
2) "When should the treatment be terminated in cases showing improvement?".   Even in
the case where vertigo has completely disappeared, if the difference between the left and
right cupulogram remains, one may predict a recurrence.   Therefore, one should continue
treatment for at least three weeks after the left-right differentiation has disappeared from
the cupulogram.   If no abnormality appears in the cupulogram during this period, treatment may be terminated.   There are many cases which show cessation of signs and symptoms while free from stress in the hospital, but show recurrence after returning to their

occupation.   Fig. 68 illustrates the case of a 34 year-old weatherman who entered the hostpial for treatment of Ménière's disease.   He returned to work shortly after being released from the hospital.   His work was in cycles of 24 hours on duty and 24 hours off duty.   Influence of the stress of his work was recorded on the cupulogram immediately before and after his work period for several months. (This is illustrated by Fig. 68.) When the patient changed to a more normal working schedule his illness remitted and he has continued in good health to the present.

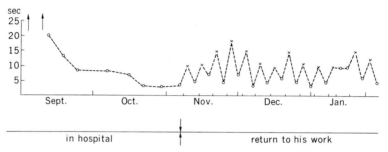

Fig. 68   Changing process of cupulogram observed in a case of Ménière's disease.
The abscissa in this graph shows difference of nystagmus duration between clockwise and counter-clockwise rotation.
o: Result of test before his work;   ×: Result of test after his work
Increase of differentiation was always observed after his work.

e. Pendular rotation test

The pendular rotation test (PR test) is different from most other rotation tests, as it is the examination of the nystagmus which is elicited during rotation, i.e. per-rotatory nystagmus.   This test was made possible by the advent of ENG, by means of which accurate recordings of per-rotatory nystagmus are possible.

The rotation test is the test for detecting a directional preponderance (DP) of nystagmus, and, at the same time, it is useful in the differential diagnosis of central and labyrinthine lesions.

There are several different pendular rotation test methods in current use; two representative methods are shown below:

i) Pendular rotation test (centric rotation)

An electrically driven pendular rotation chair is used.   The chair, shown in Fig. 69 is driven in a pendular fashion with an amplitude of 120 degrees and a period variable from 2 to 8 seconds.   The patients head is fixed at 30 degrees below the horizontal so that the lateral semicircular canals are primarily affected by the rotatory stimulus.   The input to the ocular fundus is varied by opening the eyes both with (a) and without (b) fixation on a stationary target, closing the eyes (c), and covering the eyes (d).   Eye movements are recorded by ENG.   Normal and pathological recordings are illustrated in Fig. 70.

Diagnostic Significance.   Positive findings will be obtained in cases with 1) bilateral dead labyrinths, 2) central lesions, and 3) DP.   If bilateral dead labyrinths are present no eye responses should be induced from pendular rotation with the eyes closed or covered. However, if a unilateral dead labyrinth has been present long enough for compensation to have occurred, no abnormal findings will be detectable by this test.   Cases with central lesions usually show positive findings in some of the recordings under different visual conditions.   Cases with gaze defects, for example, may show pathological record-

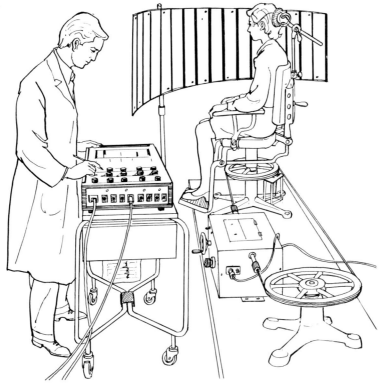

Fig. 69 Pendular rotation test.
The chair is rotated in the sinusoidal fashion with the maximum amplitude of 60 degrees.   The period
of rotation is variable from 2 to 10 seconds.   The head and the body are rotated together.

ings with the eyes open (a and b), while cases with defective inhibitory mechanisms, as
in some cerebellar lesions, may reveal findings in the recordings with the eyes closed
or covered.   D.P. will be shown in some of the recordings under different visual conditions (a,b, c, and d).

Perrotatory nystagmus is physiological nystagmus, while postrotatory nystagmus is
nystagmus which appears during recovery from an abnormally created imbalance by
rotation.   The diagnostic significance of abnormalities in each of these different kinds
of nystagmus is therefore different.

In traditional rotation tests such as cupulometry, for example, rotation must be repeated
several times with sufficiently long intervals.   When rotation is repeated, nystagmic
responses usually show a decline, and this is the greatest disadvantage of the traditional
test as a clinical tool.   Pendular rotation, however, does not elicit a response decline, as
alternating stimulation is used.

ii) Eccentric pendular rotation test

When the test subject sits away from the center of pendular rotation, the labyrinth is
exposed to both rotary and linear acceleration.   The results obtained by the eccentric
rotation test should be compared with those obtained by the ordinary pendular rotation
test.   MATSUNAGA, et al. (1968) used a pendular rotation chair which was rotated in a
pendular fashion with the amplitude of 90 degrees and period of 5 seconds.   In eccentric
rotation, the subject sat 100 cm away from the center of rotation.   According to the
report (MATSUNAGA, et al.), 15 normal subjects showed no directional preponderance (DP)

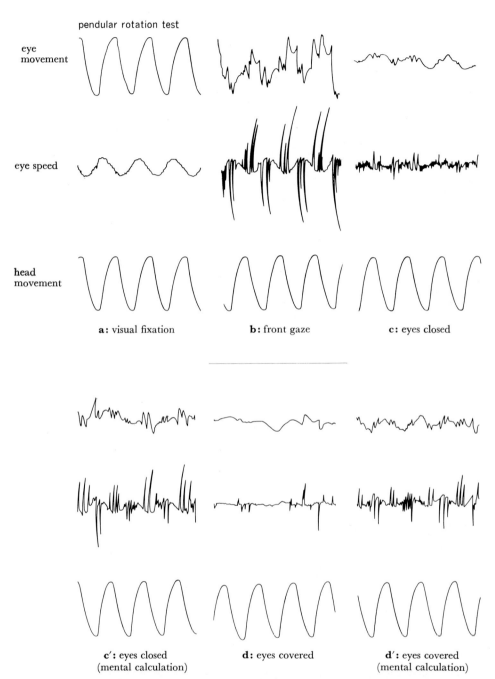

a: visual fixation   **b:** front gaze   **c:** eyes closed

c′: eyes closed   **d:** eyes covered   **d′:** eyes covered
(mental calculation)   (mental calculation)

Fig. 70   Whole-body pendular rotation test—ENG recordings from a normal subject.
The patient was instructed in (a) to maintain his gaze on a stationary target in his visual field.   In (b)
the target was removed. In (c) thru (d′) pendular rotation was continued but visual input was blocked.
Thus the only input was to the lateral canal system.   Oculomotor responses are modified by closing
or covering the eyes both with and without mental alerting.

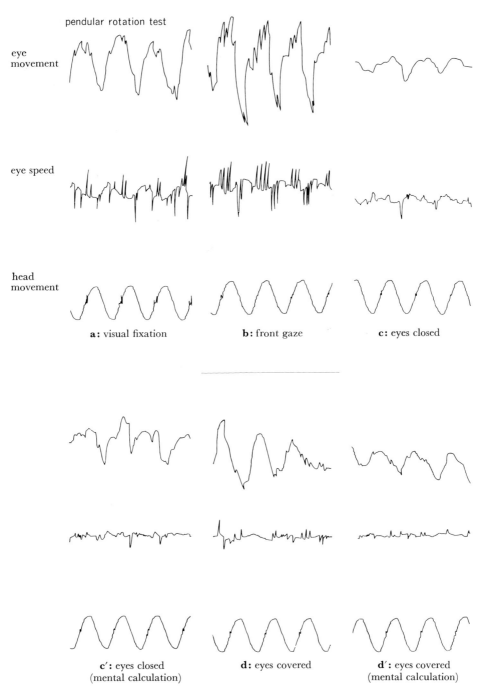

Fig. 71 a Pendular rotation test—ENG recordings from a clinical case.
Visual fixation is disturbed (a).   Large amplitude and right-left difference are noted in (b).   Irregular
eye movements can be seen in (c)–(d'), which are different from normal responses (refer to Fig. 70).

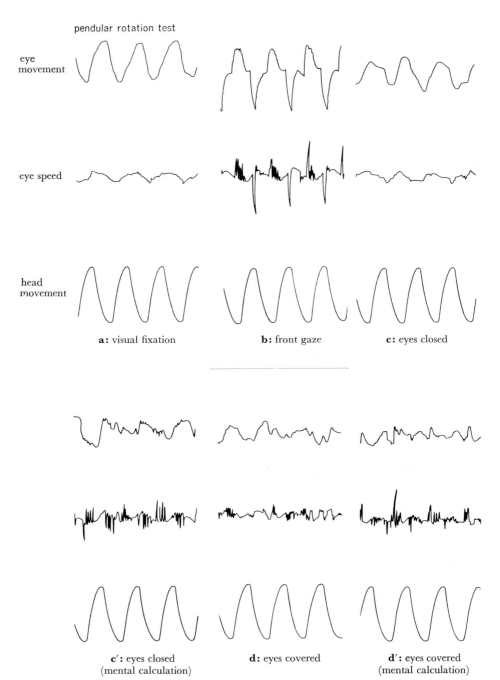

Fig. 71 b Pendular rotation test—ENG recordings from a clinical case.
Remarkable right-left differences are seen in (b). The rest of the recordings are unremarkable.

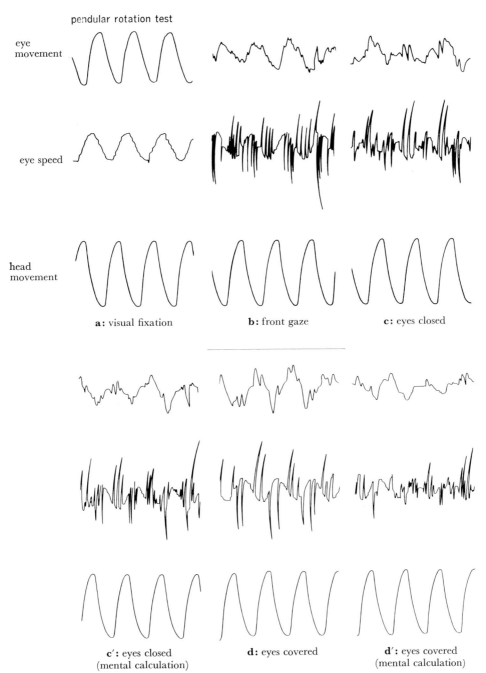

Fig. 71 c Pendular rotation test—ENG recordings from a clinical case.
Both (a) and (b) appear normal. Recordings (b) through (d′) are very similar to each other.

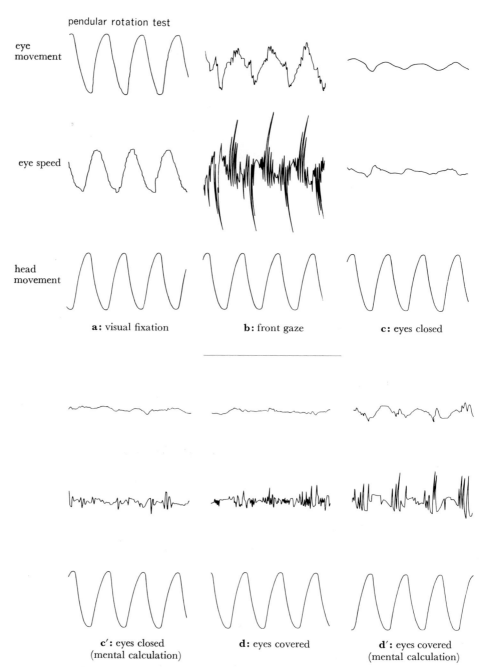

Fig. 71 d   Pendular rotation test—ENG recordings from a clinical case.
Right-left differences are seen in (d) and (d'), and only nystagmus beats to the right are noted. This may be due to the presence of a very weak spontaneous nystagmus in this case.

in nystagmus responses induced in either ordinary or eccentric pendular rotation tests. Many cases of labyrinthine lesions including Ménière's disease showed more pronounced DP in eccentric than in ordinary pendular rotation tests. This does not usually occur with cases of central lesions. The study indicates that the eccentric rotation test is useful in differentiating labyrinthine from central lesions.

f. Clinical significance of the rotation test

Some investigators are of the opinion that the rotation tests should be excluded from the list of routine vestibular tests for the following reasons:

First, with the rotation test unilateral labyrinthine reactions can not be evaluated.

Second the difference in response between the left and right labyrinth is modified by central compensation. Actually, there are some cases which show no difference in the rotatory response between the left and the right, but manifest an abnormal caloric response on one side or the other.

Third, the rotation test requires some expensive instruments. However, the rotation test should not be excluded from routine testing, for it has the following advantages: First, if the test is properly carried out, i.e. by manual cupulometry the degree of vestibular asymmetry can be precisely detected. This asymmetry varies in parallel with the severity of vertigo. Thus, the rotation test can be important for evaluating the effects of treatment. Secondly, the reversion sign of a peripheral vestibular lesion can be detected only by self-recording cupulometry. Therefore, this rotation test is valuable in differentiating peripheral vestibular disturbance from central one.

Another advantage lies in the fact that by positioning of the head various pairs of semicircular canals can be separately stimulated. Therefore, the rotation test is useful in investigating the function of not only the horizontal but also the vertical semicircular canals.

3. Test for a Labyrinthine Fistula

In certain pathologic states compression or aspiration of the air in the external auditory canal may produce nystagmus. This is known as mechanical nystagmus and was discovered by LUCAE in 1881. Usually some other vestibular reactions such as vertigo, falling etc. may accompany the nystagmus.

The most common condition demonstrating this reaction is a circumscribed defect of the bony labyrinthine capsule, i.e. a fistula with the membraneous labyrinth intact. In normal persons nystagmus does not occur when a pressure of 300 mmHg is applied (HERZOG, 1910), but when there is a fistula in the bony labyrinth it will occur with only 20 mmHg pressure (NYLÉN, 1943).

The most widely accepted theory of the mechanism of occurrence is that in the presence of a fistula in the lateral semicircular canal, positive pressure changes in the external meatus cause ampullopetal movement of the endolymphatic fluid and negative pressure changes cause its ampullofugal movement. The resultant nystagmus, according to the Ewald's law, is directed to the ipsilateral ear by compression, and to the opposite ear by aspiration. In such cases the reaction is called a typical positive reaction. If the nystagmus is of opposite nature, it is called "inverted or paradoxic positive reaction." NYLÉN (1923) explained the difference of reaction based on the underlying pathology of the fistula. If normal perilymphatic space exists between the defect in the bony wall and the membraneous labyrinth, the fistula reaction will be typical. However, if there is a direct contact between the bony defect and the membraneous labyrinth, a paradoxic fistula reaction occurs.

The test for the fistula sign is important clinically for the following reasons: mechanical nystagmus is a sign of peripheral vestibular disturbance without exception. Moreover, utilizing this test it is possible to determine the impaired side. The test is indicated in cases of vertigo with chronic otitis media to investigate whether defects of the bony labyrinthine capsule are present. Another indication for this test isgiven in cases of inner ear syphilis, particularly of the congenital form. In such cases the tympanic membranes usually appear normal and the fistular sign is often observed in spite of the absence of a demonstrable fistula. This is called the pseudofistula sign and is well known as Alexander-Hennebert's sign.

The test procedure: Usually the test is performed by using a Politzer bag. The auditory meatus must be tightly closed with the tip of the tube connected to the rubber bag, so that air can not escape. Pressure is applied to the meatus while the examiner watches for movements of the eyes or posture changes, and inquires about vertigo (Fig. 72). A sudden increase in pressure is more effective in eliciting nystagmus than a lengthy slow increase of pressure. If the examiner fails to observe nysatgmus in the initial attempt, it is probable that an immediate repeat will be unsuccessful also. The response decline phenomenon may be caused by repetition of the same stimulation; thus one should allow an adequate time to elapse between tests.

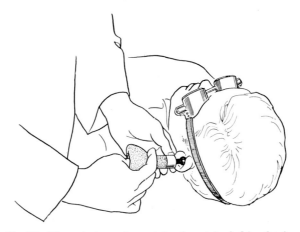

Fig. 72   The technique of examining for a labyrinthine fistula.

Nystagmus may also be observed through Frenzel glasses, but when pressure is applied to the autidory canal the patient may close his eyes because of the sudden vertigo and discomfort, and the nystagmus may be inaccessible to direct vision. If available it is preferable to use ENG for a more accurate assessment (Fig. 73 from Dr. UEMURA). Also, one can more easily elicit nystagmus if the patient is in the dorsal recumbent position with the head turned to the unimpaired side.

4.   The Galvanic Test

If one electrode is attached to the tragus and another to some part of the body (for example, the forearm) when a weak D.C. electric current is passed between their electrodes, nystagmus can be provoked. If the cathode is attached to the tragus nystagmus will occur to that side and if the anode is attached it occurs to the opposite side. This nystagmus is called galvanic nystagmus. As the mechanism causing this nystagmus still remains in dispute, there is some doubt as to whether it is possible to differentiate between labyrinthine or vestibular nerve lesions by means of the results of the galvanic test.

As seen in Fig. 74, there are four methods of electrical stimulation. With the bipolar

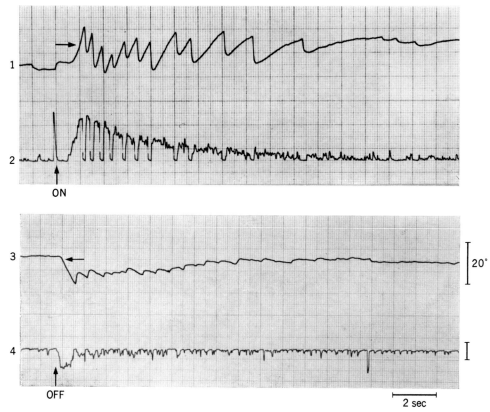

Fig. 73 A D.C. recording of a positive result of the fistula test.
The record is continuous. Lines 1 and 3 are the actual eye movements and line 2 and 4 the slow phase velocity. At the mark "on" positive air pressure was applied to the left ear canal. Note that the nystagmus began with a tonic deviation to the right or left arrows on lines 1 and 3 and that the slow phase velocity and frequency gradually declined and disappeared within 10 seconds and reappeared in the opposite direction when the pressure was released (mark "off"). The calibration for the velocity trace is 20°/sec.

binaural method one can elicit a response more easily with a weak current than with the monopolar monoaural method. However, because the binaural methods excites both ears, it is difficult to interpret the test results. The monaural method is better for detecting the function of each ear individually. Using a silver electrode of 1 cm in diameter wrapped in gauze saturated with saline solution and attached to the tragus and a plate of 10 cm × 4 cm attached to the forearm as the other electrode, nystagmus will be elicited when the

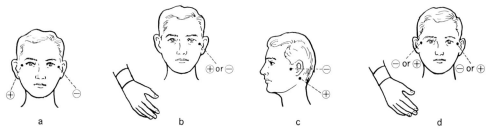

Fig. 74 Methods of electrical stimulation.
a: Bipolar binaural method; b: Unipolar uniaural method; c: Bipolar uniaural method; d: Unipolar binaural method

current is gradually increased from 1 to 6 milliamperes in normal cases.   However in some pathological cases the threshold is quite high and stimuli of more than 10 milliamperes are necessary to provoke nystagmus.   This strong current causes discomfort and pain to the patient and therefore this test should not be used in a routine examination.   However PFALTZ (1969) has developed the galvanic test using a photoelectronystagmography in which nystagmus is recorded with a much lower current, thus decreasing the pain which the patient feels and making the test usable.

Falling or tendency to fall can be also observed when galvanic stimulation is applied. FISCHER (1956) discovered that when the Mann's standing test was carried out during the bipolar biaural galvanic stimulation period, the patient tended to fall before the occurrence of nystagmus with the currents of only 1–1.5 miliamperes.   In this test the patient will not show any uncomfortable sensation.

OTOLITH FUNCTION TEST

1. Ocular Counter-rolling

When the head is tilted to the right, the eyeball will roll to the left around the line of sight and vice versa, to approximately maintain the original position of the eyeball in relation to the visual field and avoid movement of the image on the retina.   This is called counter-rolling of the eyes.   Similarly when the head is tilted forward or backward the eyeball will roll in the opposite direction either up or down: This eye movement is called vertical deviation.   These movements of the eyeball in response to a changing head position have been called compensatory counter-rolling of the eye and have been well known for many years.   In a normal person a lateral tilt of the head to 30, 45 and 60 degrees elicits an eye deviation of 4, 7 and 8.5 degrees respectively (see Fig. 75).

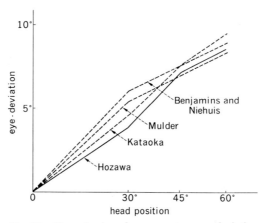

Fig. 75   Normal value of compensatory eye-deviation.

Actually compensatory ocular counter-rolling in man and other species with the eyes located in the front of the head, i.e. monkey, cat, is very incomplete as noted by the $7°$ globe rotation in response to $60°$ of body rotation.   In animals with eyes located on the sides of their heads such as rabbit or fish, these reflexes are much more complete and are also classified somewhat differently.   For example, in the rabbit rotation around the occipito-nasal axis causes vertical deviations while rotation around the bitemporal axis causes counter-rolling.   This is just opposite to animals with frontal eyes.   M.H. FISCHER (1928) showed that compensatory eye deviation derives from the labyrinth. MAGNUS (1924) thought that the cause was the change of pressure of the otolith on the macula.

Although the physiological mechanism of compensatory eye deviation has yet to be made clear in detail, the test for compensatory eye deviation may have much clinical significance: First, this test is valid for a quantitative examination of the otolith function, because it is possible to measure the tilt of the head as well as the deviation of the eye ball. Second, determination of the affected side is possible by this method. It has been demonstrated (HOZAWA, 1956) that in cases of unilateral labyrinthine hypofunction, when the patient's head was tilted to the affected side the eye deviation was less than that evoked by tilt to the normal side (Fig. 76). Thus, the side which shows less eye deviation in this test is thought to be affected side. Third, this test may be positive in patients who complain of vertigo resulting from acoustic trauma. Vertigo provoked by loud sounds is known as the Tullio's phenomenon. It has been postulated that the saccule plays some part in counter-rolling, abnormality in this test may be the first signal that the vestibular labyrinth has been injured by noise.

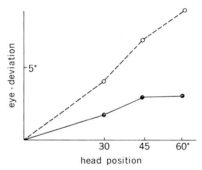

Fig. 76 Compensatory eye-deviation in a case of right acoustic tumor. When the patient's head was tilted to the right side the eye-deviation (•——•) was less than that evoked by tilt to the left side (o - - - o). This patient showed sensory-neural deafness of right ear by audiometry and right canal paresis by Hallpike's caloric test.

On the negative side, this test has the shortcoming that human counter-rolling is very small in magnitude and therefore very difficult to measure. No simple method suitable for routine clinical use has yet been developed.

In animal experiments from the time of MAGNUS it has been possible to mark a cross on the cornea and thus measure eye deviation directly. Obviously, this method can not be used with man. However various other measuring methods were devised, which can be divided into direct and indirect methods. The indirect method utilizes subjective displacement of the after-image for measurements of the eye deviation (DONDERS, 1890). This method requires highly cooperative subjects and is not as precise as the direct method. According to HOUBERT and STRUYCKEN (1925), HUECK (1838) first directly measured counterrolling of the eye by watching the conjunctival blood vessels. BÁRÁNY (1906) and KOMPANEJETZ (1923) devised special equipment for observation of eye deviation, which utilized the iris as a landmark. Furthermore, the photographic technique was applied for measuring the ocular torsion more precisely (MILLER, 1962; HOWARD and EVANS, 1963; NELSON and COPE, 1971). On the other hand, de KLEIJN and VERSTEEGH (1924) used the outer membrane from a boiled egg marked with an X placed over the conjunctiva, while BENJAMIN (1926) put two white marks with a gelatin mixture containing barium phosphate on the cornea.   Hozawa (1956) has placed small mirrors in contact lenses and used optical methods for measuring eye deviation.

These methods have several obvious drawbacks.   Direct marking of the conjunctiva may be objectionable to the patient while devises such as contact lenses placed on the cornea may move slightly in relation to the eye, thus obscuring the results.   The photographic methods are also not suitable for routine examination.   Because of the difficulty in measuring methods, compensatory eye deviation has not been widely used clinically and thus a potentially valuable tool has been neglected.   We can hope that a standardized and clinically applicable method for measuring counter-rolling will be devised in the future.

2.   Parallel Swing Test

The otolithic organs are the labyrinthine organs traditionally thought to react to linear acceleration.   When a subject is standing still, the otolithic organs detect the gravity force; if the subject moves, the reflex mechanisms work to maintain the posture erect and to hold the eyes steady in the orbits.

When the head is tilted to the side in any plane or direction the eyes deviate accordingly, usually in the opposite direction.   These eye movements are due to a reflex originating from the canals as well as from the otolithic organs.   When the head position is maintained for the minimum necessary period of time, the eyes and the body assume a specific position induced by reflex responses from the otolithic organs, and from the deep sensory receptors.

The parallel swing test is a test designed to maximally stimulate the otolithic organs and minimally stimulate the canal organs.   The plane of stimulation and the posture of the test subject can be oriented in many different positions, but the following standard position is the most practical as a clinical routine.

Method: The swing is shaped like a square or rectangular large enough to accommodate a supine adult.   The length of the ropes which hold the swing frame is limited by the height of the ceiling.   The recordings illustrated were taken from a swing which has a period of 4 sec (the length of the ropes is 282 cm), and an amplitude of 100 cm along the horizontal plane.   The subject lies supine on the swing as in Fig. 77, and is swung back and forth in the lateral direction.   During the swing movement, the subject is first asked to gaze at a point on the ceiling directly above the swing in order to calibrate the eye deviation recorded by ENG.   Eye movements are then recorded with the eyes closed and covered.

Diagnostic significance: In normal subjects, pendular eye deviation is recorded.   This is believed to be a response from the otolithic organs.   A defective response indicates bilateral otolithic afunction, and a positive response at least unilaterally normal otolithic function.

The test is useful for those cases in which standing or walking cannot be tested because of defective limb or trunk movement.   Unilateral otolithic function may not be tested by this method.   The results obtained by the test are considered together with those of the ocular counter-rotation and of the standing tests.

EXAMINATION OF EYE MOVEMENT

1.   Examination of Optokinetic Nystagmus (OKN)

When one looks out of the window of a moving train, the eyes follow the viewed objects until the extremes of the orbits are reached.   Then the eyes quickly reset and the visual following continues.   Such cyclic eye movements are called optokinetic or railroad nystagmus

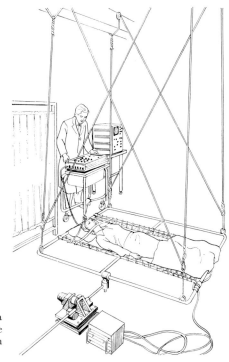

Fig. 77   Parallel swing test.
A small motor drives the swing to swing in a
sinusoidal fashion with a constant period. The
eye movements induced are recorded with an
electronystagmograph.

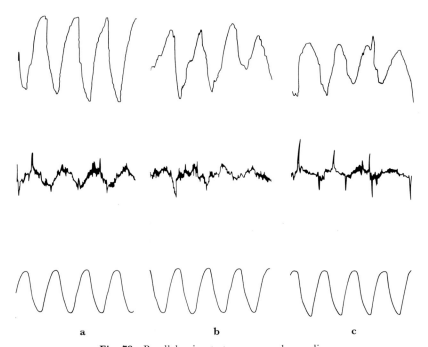

a   b   c

Fig. 78   Parallel swing test — a normal recording.
During parallel-swinging, (a) the eyes are fixed on a target, (b) the eyes are closed, and (c) the eyes are
open and covered.   The top recordings are eye movements, the second, eye speed, and the bottom,
movements of the swing.

By following moving targets with the eyes visual acquity is improved as the visual images are stablized on the retina. Optokinetic stimulation induces nystagmus and this mechanism undoubtedly helps our visual recognition of moving targets. Human subjects have active eye movements and optokinetic responses.* In certain disease states with lesions in the central nervous system OKN is definitely abnormal. In patients with brainstem lesions, for example, OKN responses are usually markedly depressed and show a great variation depending on the site and the extent of the lesions. These facts justify the introduction of the OKN examination into the clinic for diagnostic purposes.

Method. Traditionally neurologists used a tape measure for eliciting and examining OKN (Fig. 79). This method is useful for diagnosing severe or extensive defects in OKN. The introduction into the clinic of an electrically driven rotating drum as an optokinetic stimulator, and an electronystagmograph as a recorder of both eye movements and eye speed had made the OKN examination highly quantitative and definitely increased its diagnostic value (Fig. 80).

The most important features of the modern OKN examination procedure are summarized as follows:

1)   Quantitative stimulation should be given to the test subject. The OKN stimulator to be selected is a large optokinetic drum (Ohm type) with electrically controlled velocity and acceleration.**

2)   Quantitative and simultaneous recordings of both eye movements and eye speed are important. This is conveniently accomplished by using an electronystagmograph. Using this instrument one can accurately determine eye speed, nystagmus frequency, and the direction of the quick phases of the induced nystagmus.

The feeding speed of the recording chart can be as fast as 10–30 mm/sec in order to accurately measure slow phase eye speed from the eye movement recording. By slowing the feeding speed to 0.5–1.0 mm/sec, changes in the slow phase eye speed may be conveniently demonstrated.

a. Optokinetic pattern test (OKP test)

This is one of the most popular methods for testing optokinetic eye responses. With this test method, the eye speed recording is condensed by slowing the feeding speed of the chart and the recording is then seen as a pattern which simply indicates three important characteristics of the responses: 1) the direction, 2) the increase in slow phase eye speed, and 3) the frequency of the induced optokinetic nystagmus.

1)   Stimulation is applied as follows: a standard*** drum 90 cm high, 180 cm in diameter, with 12 black stripes each 2.5 cm wide equally spaced on the white background inside the drum, is rotated with a constant acceleration of $4°/sec^2$ up to a maximum velocity of 160–180°/sec, and then decelerated, with a deceleration of $-4°/sec^2$, to a standstill. The drum is first rotated counterclockwise, and then clockwise.

2)   Recording of the eye responses is performed as follows: optokinetic nystagmus is recorded with a long time constant (1.0–6.0 seconds or more; eye movement record) and with a short time constant (0.01–0.03 seconds; velocity record) simultaneously. The chart feeding speed is 0.1 cm per second to give OKP (Fig. 81) and 1.0–3.0 cm per second

---

  * OKN in some animals is as good but usually animal OKN is inferior to that of humans.
 ** For diagnostic purposes, the maximum drum-speed is usually set between 120–200 deg/sec. In normal subjects, the eyes can follow the stripes as fast as a quarter of a rotation a second or 90 degrees per second. The maximum velocity of the slow phase eye speed during OKN shows a relatively large individual variation, however.
*** A standard drum of these specifications was used, however drums of other sizes may work equally well.

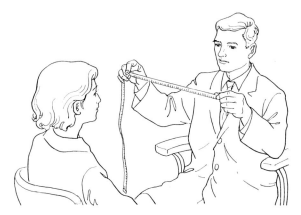

Fig. 79 Optokinetic nystagmus examination with a tape measure.
The simple procedure is useful for detecting remarkable depression, asymmetry, or inversion in optokinetic responses.

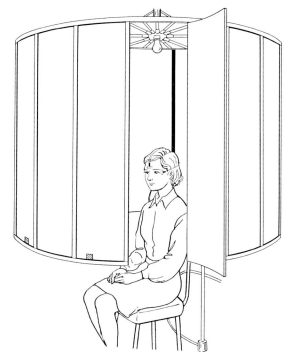

Fig. 80 A stimulator for inducing optokinetic eye responses — an optokinetic drum after Ohm.
The speed and the acceleration of the drum rotation is electrically controlled.

for analyzing individual nystagmus patterns. The OKP obtained by counterclockwise drum rotation is called right-OKP, and the one from clockwise rotation, left-OKP, since the quick phase of induced nystagmus is directed to the right in the former, and to the left in the latter.

b. Normal and abnormal findings in the OKP test

1) The direction of the quick phase of OKN in normal subjects is the opposite of the drum rotation. Abnormal responses can be elicited in the opposite direction to this, i.e.

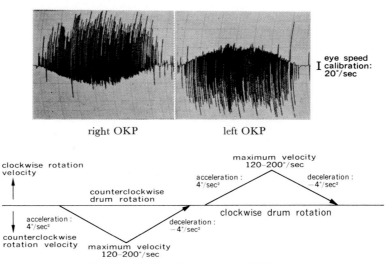

Fig. 81   Optokinetic pattern test (OKP).
A normal OKP and the method of drum rotation.

in the direction of drum rotation (inversive response) and/or can occur to both the right and left with unidirectional stimulation.

2)   The slow phase eye speed in normal subjects increases along with the increase in drum speed up to about 90°/sec. The maximum slow phase eye speed is usually not much more or less than 100°/sec. The middle portion of the OKP response is different in different individuals and even in normal subjects can be flat, convex or concave. There may be slight but very little variation between right and left OKPs in normal subjects (Fig. 81).

3)   The frequency of induced nystagmus is expressed in the OKP as density changes. The middle parts of the OKP usually have the highest density in normal subjects, nystagmic beats being about 4 per second. A density lower or a higher than this in the central portions of the response usually indicates an abnormal response.

c.   **Diagnostic significance of optokinetic nystagmus**

1)   Optokinetic nystagmus is believed to be caused by a function of the oculomotor system which favors the subjects recognition of moving targets. This is primarily a reflex response but is also strongly influenced by the will and state of alertness. Definite disturbances in the OKN responses usually indicate lesions within the oculomotor or visual system.

2)   The influences on the OKN responses from systems other than the oculomotor system are less intensive when compared to those of the oculomotor system. For example, a unilateral lesion in the labyrinth which belongs to the vestibular system has no substantial influence on optokinetic nystagmus. Fig. 84 shows the OKP from a case of Ménière's disease with spontaneous nystagmus to the right. There is a difference between the right and the left OKPs, i.e., in the middle portion of OKPs, the right OKP has higher top (due to the elevated slow phase eye speed during high speed drum rotation) and higher density (due to the higher frequency of nystagmus) compared to the left OKP.

3)   The cerebellum appears to have a significant influence on the OKP response. Some characteristic OKPs obtained from cases with cerebellar diseases are shown in Fig. 85. They may be influenced by additional lesions in the brainstem which are difficult to indentify. They are characterized by a markedly depressed slow phase eye speed and by a depressed and usually constant infrequent frequency of nystagmus.

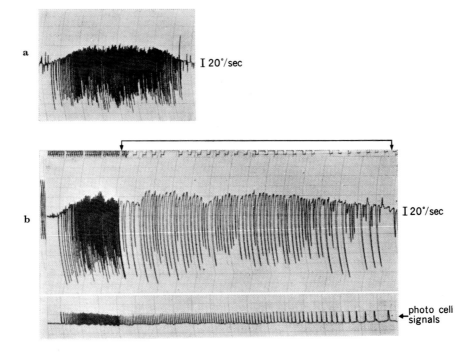

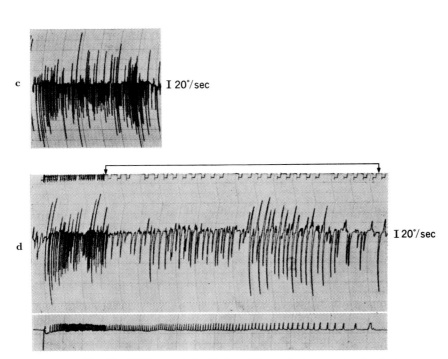

Fig. 82 OKPs recorded with two different feeding speeds of a chart.
(a) and (b) are from a normal test subject. In (b), the second part of the recording was recorded at
0.5cm/sec($\downarrow$——$\downarrow$), while the first part was recorded at 0.1cm/sec. Recordings in (c) and (d) are from
a clinical case with brainstem lesions. The method of recording in (d) is the same as in (b).

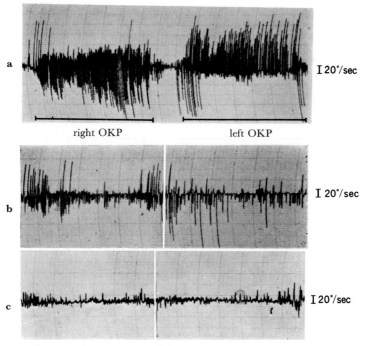

Fig. 83   OKPs — three clinical cases with unusual quick phases.

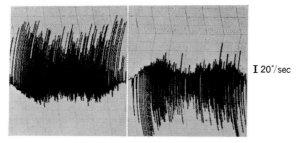

Fig. 84   An OKP — Ménière's disease.
This appears normal except for an asymmetry between the right- and the left OKPs.

4) Some parts of the brainstem appear to have much more significant influences on OKN than other parts. Changes in OKP or OKN due to brainstem lesions appear to be entirely different depending on the site of the lesion. This indicates the possibility of detailed local diagnosis as revealed by the OKN examination.

Typical OKPs obtained from clinical cases are shown in Fig. 87; a marked depression in only the middle portions of both pairs of OKPs is frequently encountered in cases of cerebellar pontine angle lesions; marked depression of the whole OKP response and a loss of the directionality of nystagmus are usually seen in pontine lesions.

5) Spontaneous nystagmus due to lesions in the visual or oculomotor system (acquired or congenital) usually gives characteristic OKPs (Fig. 86), and the OKN test frequently provides information valuable in distinguishing these lesions. Spontaneous nystagmus in these cases usually has a distinct appearance, but this is not always true especially when the nystagmus is jerking in type. OKP is especially useful in differentiating these specific spontaneous nystagmus complexes from others, such as vestibular or cerebellar nystagmus.

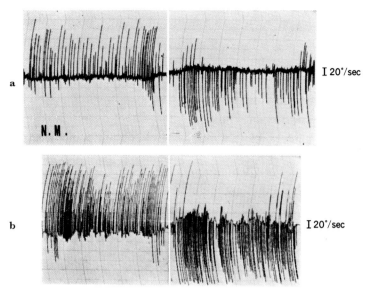

Fig. 85 OKPs — two clinical cases with cerebellar lesions.

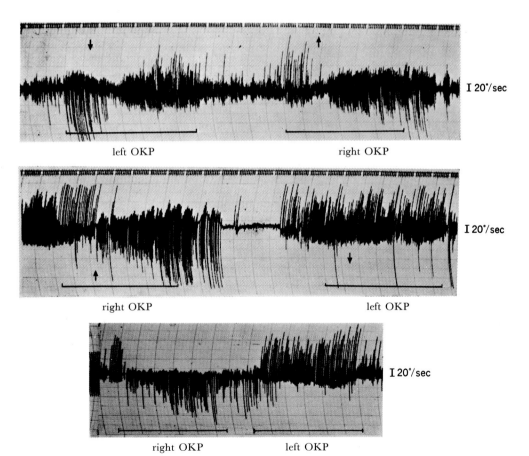

Fig. 86 OKPs — three clinical cases of congenital nystagmus.

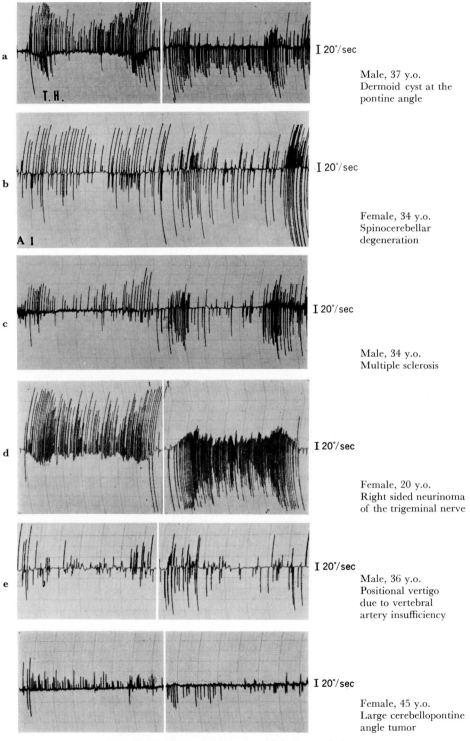

a   I 20°/sec

Male, 37 y.o.
Dermoid cyst at the
pontine angle

b   I 20°/sec

Female, 34 y.o.
Spinocerebellar
degeneration

c   I 20°/sec

Male, 34 y.o.
Multiple sclerosis

d   I 20°/sec

Female, 20 y.o.
Right sided neurinoma
of the trigeminal nerve

e   I 20°/sec

Male, 36 y.o.
Positional vertigo
due to vertebral
artery insufficiency

I 20°/sec

Female, 45 y.o.
Large cerebellopontine
angle tumor

Fig. 87   OKPs — clinical cases with brainstem lesions.

2. Examination of optokinetic after-nystagmus (OKAN)

When optokinetic stimulation is suddenly terminated after a sufficiently long period of stimulation, after-nystagmus is usually provoked for a limited length of time in darkness. This is frequently followed by the secondary phase of after-nystagmus. Optokinetic after-nystagmus occurs in the same direction as optokinetic nystgmus, and the secondary phase, in the opposite direction. If OKN is absent, OKAN will obviously be absent. The after-nystagmus appears to be closely related to the directional preponderance of the nystagmus (DP), which indicates a tonic imbalance within the central nervous system. OKAN which is prominent in the monkey was reduced to both sides, ipsilateral more than contralateral, after unilateral labyrinthectomy, and was abolished by bilateral labyrinthectomy (UEMURA and COHEN, 1972). This suggests that the vestibular labyrinth plays an important role in maintaining OKAN.

Method. To compare after-nystagmus in the two directions, right and left, the optokinetic stimulation which mobilizes after-nystagmus should be quantitatively equal bilaterally. To insure equivalent optokinetic stimulation bilaterally as an effective stimulus for inducing OKAN the original OKN must be carefully inspected. The slow phase eye speed, and the frequency of induced nystagmus are utilized for comparing the

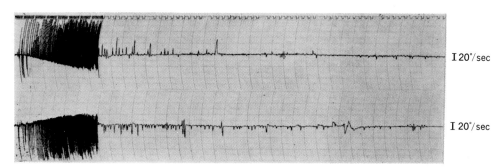

I 20°/sec

I 20°/sec

Fig. 88 Optokinetic after-nystagmus.

right and the left OKN responses. A drum of the Ohm type is best utilized since it is most powerful in inducing nystagmus. A set of OKN to the right and to the left is examined and the maximum drum speed is found which induces the same amount of OKN response in either direction, since the maximum OKN responses to the two sides are often different. To find the proper drum speed to test for OKAN the drum is accelerated in either direction until the OKN response reaches a maximum (Fig. 88). The drum speed to be selected is the one which evokes the maximum response in the less responsive direction.

For OKAN examination, the drum is rotated with 1°/sec acceleration up to the maximum speed indicated by the above "pre-test", and then, the stimulation is suddenly stopped by completely darkening the room or by covering the eyes. The eyes are kept open during OKAN recording. The simultaneous recording of OKAN and eye velocity (2 channels) is usually performed at a chart speed 0.5–1.0 cm per second. The test is completed by repeating the drum rotation in the opposite direction.

Diagnostic significance. After-nystagmus is usually evaluated by measuring its duration and frequency. After-nystagmus to the right and to the left are compared. A significant directional difference or prepondcrance (DP) indicates a central imbalance. The DP which is revealed by the OKAN test may be called "visual DP", i.e., evoked by visual stimulation in contrast to the "vestibular DP", which is evoked by vestibular stimulation.

In humans, OKAN is present with the eyes closed, covered and in complete darkness, but is usually absent with the eyes open in the light.   Recording of OKAN for clinical purposes is best done with the eyes open and covered, as active OKAN is usually maximized in this condition.   OKAN recorded with the eyes closed is usually less active or different from OKAN with the eyes covered; therefore, the visual condition must be noted, whenever the examination is performed.

3.   Eye-Tracking (ET) Test

Visual acquity is maximum when the images fall directly on the fovea.   When visual targets move, the eyes must follow the targets in order to hold the images on the fovea. This is one of the fundamental functions of the oculomotor system and is extremely important if the eyes are to accurately resolve moving targets.

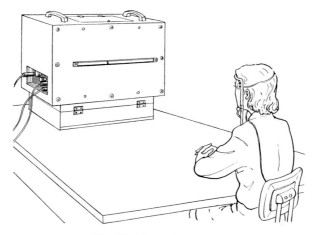

Fig. 89   Eye-tracking test.
The small visual target makes sinusoidal movements in the horizontal or in the vertical planes.

Optokinetic responses may be obtained in lower animals such as birds, or even rabbits and crabs, which do not have foveal vision, however, eye tracking is most prominent in animals with foveal vision and one of the most prominent features of the oculomotor system in animals which have binocular and foveal vision, i.e. man and higher monkeys. A test to examine the above following function is called the eye tracking test.

Method.   A target, which is clearly defined on the background, is usually moved in a sinusoidal fashion, in the horizontal direction and, when needed, also in the vertical direction.   The period is usually set between 2–6 seconds.   The head is held motionless and eye movements and speed are recorded by an electronystagmograph.

Diagnostic significance.   In normal eye tracking, both the eye movement and velocity records are smooth (Fig. 90).   This is true for eye tracking within a visual angle of 20–30 degrees with a period of 3–5 seconds.

When a patient has spontaneous nystagmus, nystagmic beats are frequently, but not always, superimposed on the smooth eye tracking curve in the direction of the spontaneous nystagmus.   Cases with lesions in the brainstem or in the cerebellum frequently show saccadic eye movements superimposed upon their smooth pursuit eye movements (Fig. 91). The degree of saccadazation present is different in each case.   Namely, the steps during the course of eye movement from one lateral extreme to the other can be rough, 2–3 steps,

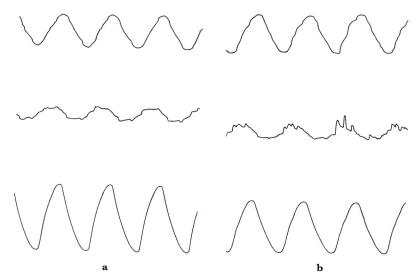

Fig. 90 Eye-tracking test — a normal and a clinical case.
The top recording is eye movements, the second, eye speed, the bottom, target motion. (a) recording from a normal subject. (b) recording from a case of Ménière's disease. In (b), there are saccadic movements only to the right superimposed on a fairly smooth tracking motion of the eyes.

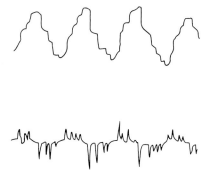

Fig. 91 Eye-tracking test — a clinical case of brainstem lesion.
Rough saccades replace smooth sinusoidal eye-tracking seen in normal subjects. Saccades are seen in both the right and left directions, different from the saccades in Fig. 90 b where they are only unidirectional.

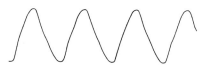

or fine, 7–8 steps. Course steps usually indicate a more severe dysfunction than do fine steps. These saccadic eye movements are clearly shown as spikes in the eye speed recording as shown in Fig. 91. As demonstrated in Fig. 92A, atactic pursuit is sometimes seen in cerebellar cases. Again, the degree of ataxia can be marked or slight. It should be emphasized that electronystagmographic recording is the most accurate and readily

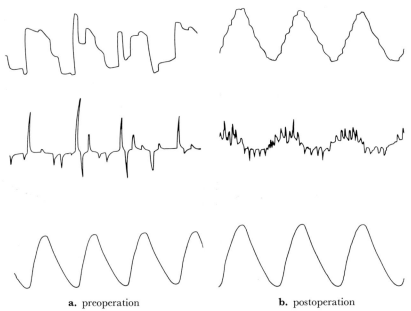

a. preoperation   **b.** postoperation

Fig. 92 A   Eye-tracking test, two recordings before and after extirpation of a right sided acoustic
            neurinoma.
(a) the recording before operation is atactic rather than saccadic and (b) the one after operation is
saccadic.   These saccades are finer than those in Fig. 91.

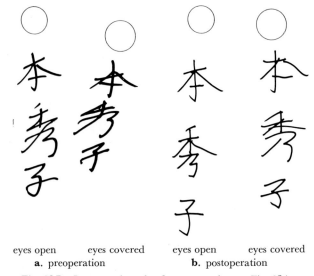

eyes open   eyes covered   eyes open   eyes covered
          a. preoperation   **b.** postoperation

Fig. 92 B   Letters written by the same patient as Fig. 92A.

available method for recording the ataxia found by this test. This finding should be
compared with the ataxia in the limbs, which is usually observed visually and is not
usually so accurately recorded as that of the eyes.

In the OKN test, at least in humans, both peripheral and foveal retinal images are con
cerned with mobilizing the eyes, but in the ET test, only foveal images are brought into play.
Abnormal results of the OKN and the ET tests, accordingly, have a different diagnostic

significance.   Both tests are under the control of the visuo-oculomotor reflexes or involuntary mental influences, but also are intensively influenced by the will.   The reflex controls and voluntary influences on OKN and ET are, however, different.

Evaluation of the Autonomic Nervous System

It has been assumed for many years that disturbance of the blood supply to the labyrinth could be the cause of Ménière's disease.   In 1922 KOBRAK advocated that Ménière's disease should be renamed "angioneurotic crisis".   LERMOYEZ (1929) put forward the theory that an ischemia of the labyrinth due to spasm of the internal auditory artery or its branches could be the cause of the vestibular and cochlear symptoms.   Later, this presumed spasm of the internal auditory artery or its branches, or both was widely conceived as being part of a generalized imbalance of the vasoconstrictor and vasodilator functions of the autonomic nervous system.   Thus tests of the autonomic nervous system are often essential for evaluating the causes of vertigo.   Blood pressure is routinely evaluated in vertigo cases.   SAKATA (1964) observed that aural vertigo such as Ménière's disease, positional vertigo of the benign paroxysmal type and sudden deafness were commonly accompanied by hypotonia.   Hypotonia often creates an area of dysfunction in the labyrinth secondary to anoxia, and seems to be a predisposing condition for vertigo. Standard tests for the evaluation of the autonomic nervous system have not been established.   For this purpose we recommend observing the changes on blood pressure evoke by DRESEL's epinephrine test or the methacholine chloride test.

1. DRESEL's Epinephrine Test

A 1: 1000 solution of epinephrine is injected subcutaneously in a dose of 0.13 ml per 10 kg of body weight. Brachial blood pressure is measured before the injection and every 2 minutes after the injection for the first 10 minutes and then every 10 minutes for the next 50 minutes.   The value of blood pressure is graphed; the abscissa is the time after injection in minutes, the ordinate, the value of blood pressure in mmHg.   As seen in Fig. 93, there are three types of curves indicating the blood pressure changes caused by epinephrine injection.   The first shows a peak between ten and twenty minutes and then gradually declines to normal (type A).   The second climbs rapidly, peaking within ten minutes, and then declines rapidly.   This indicates a sympathetic hyperreactor (type B).   The third peaks late and declines slowly.   This indicates sympathetic hyporeactor (type C). Among 27 cases of Ménière's diseases tested by this method, only 4 cases were normal; most cases showed type B or C.   It was also shown that the results are not influenced by the physical condition at the time of testing, i.e. in the same patient, as seen in Fig. 94 the type of the blood pressure curve tested in the morning on an empty stomach was identical with that taken in the evening after bathing and eating.

2. Methacholine Chloride Test

This test was devised by FUNKENSTEIN et al. (1948).   GELHORN and REDGATE (1955) observed the fact that decline of blood pressure induced by methacholine chloride injection stimulated the sympathetic autonomic centers and consequently the rise in blood pressure was provoked.   They proposed that by investigating the changes in blood pressure hypothalamic sympathetic excitability could be evaluated.

This test is performed by the following procedure: Methachloine chloride is injected intramuscularly in a dose of 10 mg per 60 kg of body weight.   After injection, brachial blood pressure is measured every 30 seconds for the first 5 minutes and then every 1

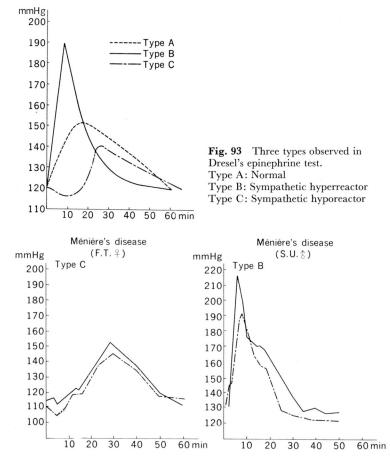

Fig. 93 Three types observed in Dresel's epinephrine test.
Type A: Normal
Type B: Sympathetic hyperreactor
Type C: Sympathetic hyporeactor

Fig. 94 The influence of the physical condition at the time of testing on the blood pressure curve.
The result tested in the morning on empty stomach (broken line) was identical with that in the evening after having a bath (black line).

minute for the next 20 minutes. The value of systolic blood pressure is graphed. The abscissa is the time after injection (1 min. = 1 cm), and the ordinate is the value of blood pressure (5 mmHg = 1 cm). The area between the ascending limb of the blood pressure curve and the line parallel to the abscissa from the point indicating the bottom value of blood pressure is measured and is divided by the maximum fall of the blood pressure. The quotient, which is termed the Mecholyl Index (M.I.), can be differentiated into three types; sympathetic hyperreactor when M.I. is over 3.76, intermediate group or normoreactor when M.I. is between 2.09 and 3.76, and sympathetic hyporeactor when M.I. is below 2.09. From the result of repeated Mecholyl tests during the course of Ménière's disease, UEMURA et al. (1972) have reported that abnormalities in the autonomic nervous system are related to the cause of the disease and are not merely a reflection of the vertiginous episode.

It was noted that no matter whether Dresel's test or the methacholine chloride test was used in testing the same person, the results were nearly equivalent. It may be concluded that the examination of the curve derived from blood pressure changes provoked by a stimulus is an appropriate method for detecting the autonomic dystonia which may under-lie the vertiginous condition.

X-ray Studies

The diagnostic value of the roentgenologic examination in the field of neuro-otology is invaluable. For example, organic change of the labyrinth may sometimes be well detected by radiographs of the temporal bone, the diagnosis of acoustic tumor is usually finally decided by X-ray studies, the origin of cervical vertigo is documented by projections of the cervical vertebrae or vertebral angiography, and intracranial lesions causing central vestibular disturbance can often be revealed by pneumoventriculography or angiography. Several routine methods of X-ray examination used in the field of neuro-otology will now be reviewed.

1. Roentgenography of the Petrous Portion (Labyrinth) of the Temporal Bone
STENVERS' projection

In this projection, the patient is prone, the head is turned 45 degrees toward the side being radiographed and the chin is flexed bringing the orbito-meatal lines into the vertical position. This makes the axis of the pyramid horizontal. In this projection, the petrous apex, the petrous ridge, the internal auditory canal, the anterior and lateral semicircular canals and the vestibule are well shown (Fig. 95). The region of the cochlea can

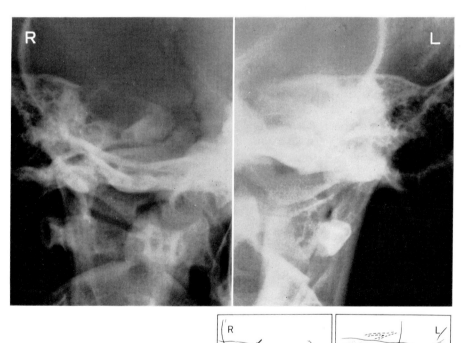

Fig. 95 STENVERS' projection.
Left (L): Normal
Right (R): Destruction of the pyramis for acoustic neurinoma.

be delineated, but its finer detail is not apparent.   There are very narrow limits for the correct positioning of the head for this projection, i.e. incorrect head position results in the superimposition of the shadows of other bone structures upon the petrous portion of the temporal bone (Fig. 96).   A clear picture will be impossible unless the angle of the head and the X-ray beam are exactly aligned.   One can anticipate good results if a fluoroscope can be used for aiming before taking the radiograph.

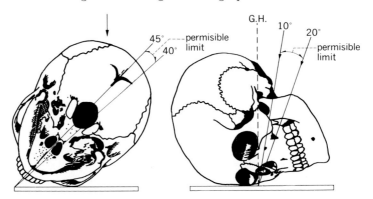

Fig. 96   The correct positioning of the head for STENVERS' projection. G.H.: German horizontal (tangential to the inferior orbital rims and the upper margins of the external auditory meati).

This method has diagnostic value in cases of acoustic tumor.   STENVERS has proposed the following classification for cases of acoustic tumor.

a)   Those in which the internal auditory canal is enlarged or in which there is only minor destruction of the pyramis.

b)   Those in which the internal auditory canal is normal, but with extensive destruction of the pyramis.

c)   Those in which there is deformation of the medial-inferior part of the pyramis.

STENVERS' projection is also useful in determining the presence of a pyramis fracture and is very important in detecting labyrinthine fracture in cases of head injury.

2.   Roentgenography of the Internal Auditory Canals

In STENVERS' projection, it is impossible to take an X-ray photograph of both internal auditory canals at the same time.   In order to precisely compare the size of the left and right canals, it is very helpful to have simultaneous bilateral projections.   It is reported (EPISTEIN, 1950) that in only 2 cases of 15, internal auditory canal enlargement could be detected using STENVERS' projection, however in 6 out of 19 this finding was revealed by TOWNE's projection.

a.   TOWNE's projection

The patient lies supine, facing the X-ray tube with the head flexed and the chin depressed so that the orbito-meatal line lies perpendicular to the film.   The central ray is angled 32 degrees caudally and directed along the median sagittal plane to pass through the intermeatal plane to the center of the film.

Since both internal auditory canals are demonstrated on one film and can be directly compared, it is possible to evaluate whether one side is enlarged or not.   Especially, as TOWNE (1926) pointed out, a funnel shape on the affected side as compared to the normal side is a clear indication of the presence of a tumor (see Fig. 97).

In this projection, the permissible limits of the projection angle of the internal auditory

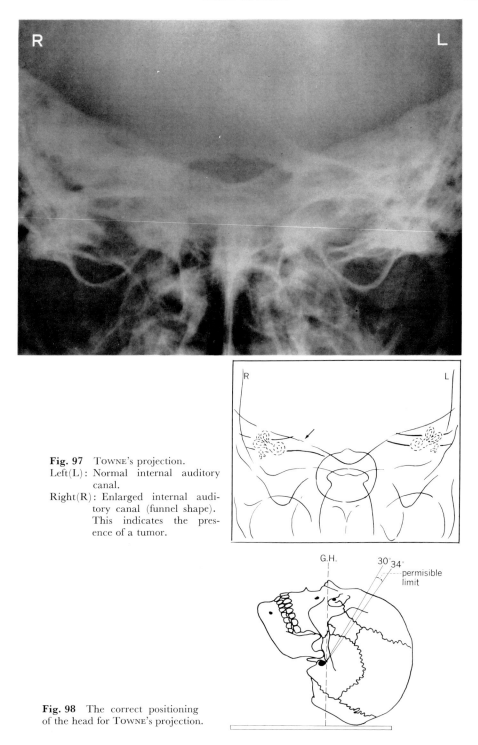

Fig. 97 TOWNE's projection.
Left(L): Normal internal auditory canal.
Right(R): Enlarged internal auditory canal (funnel shape). This indicates the presence of a tumor.

Fig. 98 The correct positioning of the head for TOWNE's projection.

canals to exclude the superimposition of the shadows of other bone structures are very narrow (Fig. 98). This is an effective method for radiography when a fluoroscope is used for aiming the X-ray beam.

b. Antero-posterior projection through the orbits

The patient lies supine facing the tube.   The orbito-meatal line is depressed 7–10 degrees and central ray is directed to the median sagittal plane and the interpupillary plane to the center of the film.   This view projects the internal auditory meati through the orbits and allows comparison of the two sides on one film (Fig. 99).

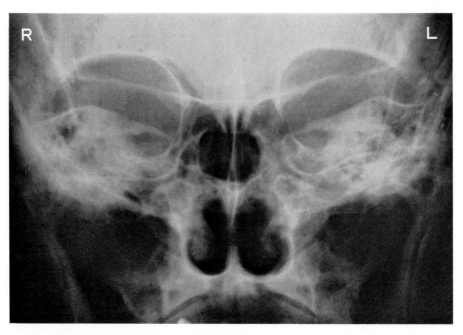

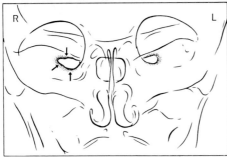

Fig. 99   Antero-posterior projection through the orbits.
This view projects the internal auditory meati through the orbits and allows comparison of the two sides on one film.
R: Tumor side   L: Normal side

c. Circus tomography of the internal auditory canal

Circus tomography is useful in obtaining a clear picture of the internal auditory canal, especially in Towne's position it gives good anatomical detail of the canal, as shown in Fig. 100.   This method is very useful for the early diagnosis of acoustic tumor.

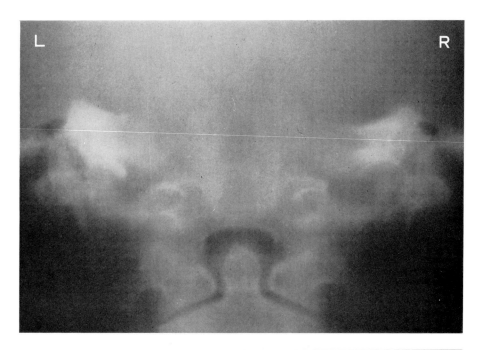

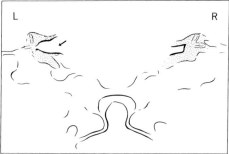

Fig. 100   Circus tomography of the internal auditory canal.
R: Tumor side   L: Normal side

3. Roentgenography of the Mastoid and Tympanic Cavities

SCHÜLLER's projection is a sort of lateral projection of the temporal bone. To avoid superimposition on the opposite temporal bone, the cranial eccentric lateral projection is employed. This projection is used for study of the mastoid. The mastoid process is projected posterior to the posterior surface of the petrous pyramid, the squama and the zygomatic region are observed by this method (Fig. 101).

The tympanic region can be demonstrated by MAYER's projection. In this projection, the patient is supine, the head is rotated 45 degrees toward the side being radiographed

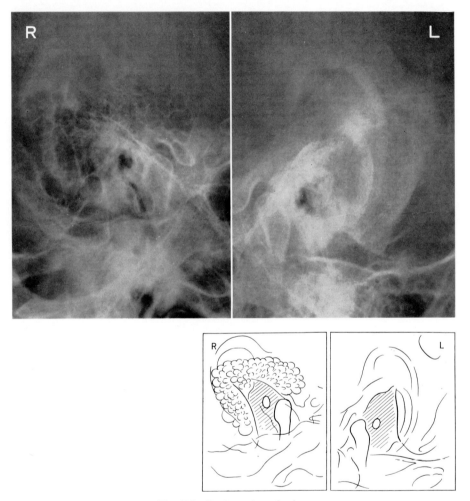

Fig. 101 SCHÜLLER's projection.

and is flexed so that the orbito-meatal line becomes vertical. The X-ray beam is tilted 45 degrees cranial eccentric.

This projects the petrous portion away from the tympanic region and its vicinity, so that there is a minimum superimposition of heterogeneous structures upon the mastoid antrum, the aditus ad antrum, the tympanic cavity and the external auditory canal (Fig. 102).

SCHÜLLER's and MAYER's projections can indicate the position of the sigmoid sinus which is of great importance in labyrinthine surgery.

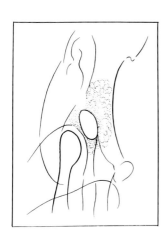
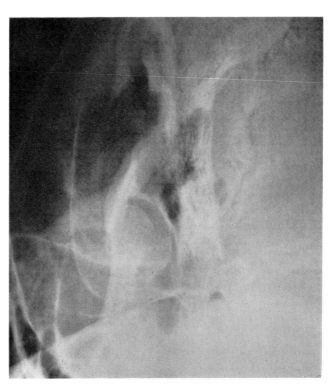

Fig. 102 MAYER's projection.

4. Roentgenography of the Skull

Three projection methods of the skull are routinely used in cases of head injury.

In order to find the extent of the fracture, bitemporal, fronto-occipital and submento-vertical projections are routinely employed.

Because of individual variations, one must take special care in evaluating the roentgenogram of the base of skull. In this projection, the shape of internal auditory canal, foramina magnum and foramina jugulare are evaluated.

5. Roentgenography of the Cervical Spine and Intervertebral Foramina

This method provides suggestive evidence for the diagnosis of the cervicovestibular syndrome and vertebral-basilar insufficiency. Since deformation of the cervical spine usually occurs at $C_{4\,5\,6}$, it is sufficient to take a lateral as well as ventro-dorsal view focusing on C_5 (Fig. 103). Also, there is often a narrowing of the foramina intervertebrale which can be detected by roentgenography (Fig. 104).

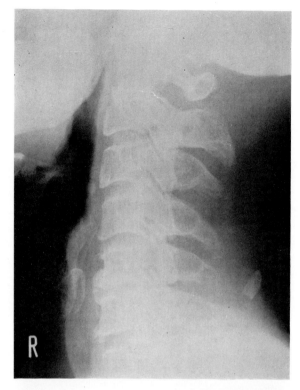

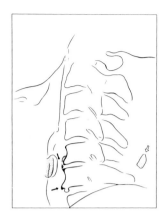

Fig. 103 Roentgenography of the cervical spine.
Deformation of the cervical spine (C$_{5, 6}$) (↓) and Barsony's calcification (↻) can be observed.

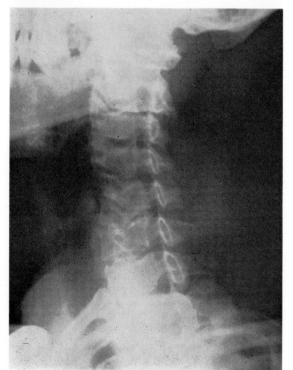

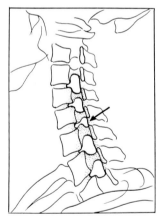

Fig. 104 Roentgenography of the intervertebral foramina.

Roentgenography of the second cervical vertebra is a most effective method for diagnosing basilar impression. When the processus vermiformis is higher than a horizontal line drawn between the two incisura mandibulae one should suspect basilar impression.

6. Angiography

Carotid angiography (CAG) and vertebral angiography (VAG) are often employed in the field of neuro-otology. Specifically in cases of cervicovestibular syndrome and vertebral-basilar insufficiency, the findings revealed by VAG are very imporatnt (Fig. 105). Abnormal findings such as malformation, abnormal shift, obstruction, narrowing, kinking, sclerosis and aneurysm etc. are often observed with angiography.

There are various methods of angiography. We routinely inject 10 ml of 60% Conray directly into the vertebral artery or into a SELDINGER catheter threaded centrally from the right brachial artery when photographing the right vertebral artery, and into the right femoral artery when photographing the left side.

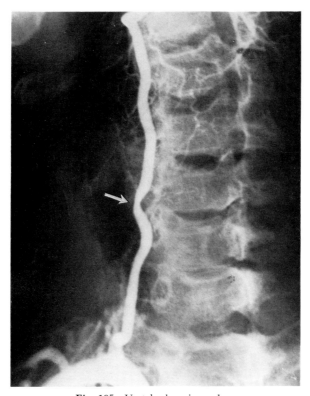

Fig. 105 Vertebral angiography.
Narrowing ($\rightarrow$) of vertebral artery is observed in a case of cervicovestibular syndrome.

7. Pantopaque Cisternography and Pneumoencephalography

A recent technique in which a small amount of pantopaque is placed into the subdural space at the lumbar level and then by changing the position of the patient is manipulated into the cerebellopontine angle has been described. By this method the internal

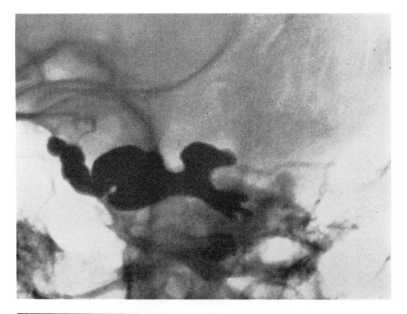

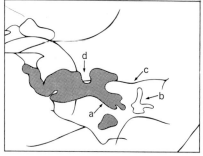

a. Internal auditory canal
b. Labyrinth
c. Arcuate eminence
d. Notch caused by the trigeminal nerve
e. Acoustic tumor

A. Normal internal auditory canal outlined by the contrast material.

Fig. 106 Pantopaque cisternography.
(Courtesy of Dr. N. KOBAYASHI, Associate Professor of Neuroradiology, Tokyo Women's Medical College.)

auditory meatus can be filled with contrast material and small cerebellopontine angle tumors well delineated (Fig. 106). Pneumoencephalography may also be useful for the purpose of demonstrating certain congenital anomalies and conditions associated with atrophy of the brain (Fig. 107). A controlled PEG is important in detecting subtentorial lesion (Fig. 108). Specifically, combined PEG and circus tomography is very useful for early diagnosis of acoustic tumor, as shown in Fig. 109.

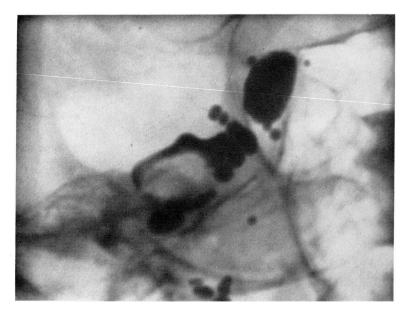

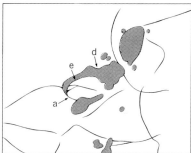

B. Acoustic tumor outlined protruding from the internal auditory canal.

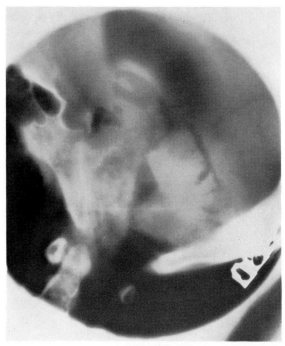

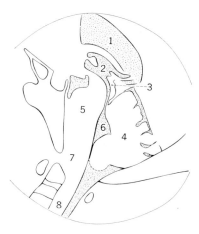

1. Lateral ventricle
2. Third ventricle
3. Corpora quadrigemina
4. Cerebellum
5. Pons
6. Fourth ventricle
7. Medulla oblongata
8. Spinal cord

A.   Normal pneumoencephalogram — a midline laminogram.

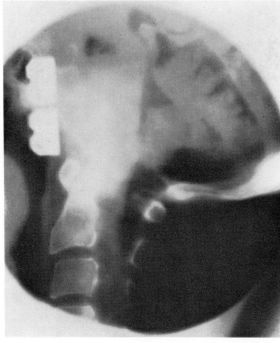

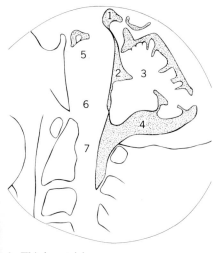

1. Third ventricle
2. Fourth ventricle
3. Cerebellum
4. Cisterna magnum
5. Pons
6. Medulla oblongata
7. Spinal cord

B.   Cerebellar atrophy — thin cerebellar folia combined with dilated cisterna magnum.

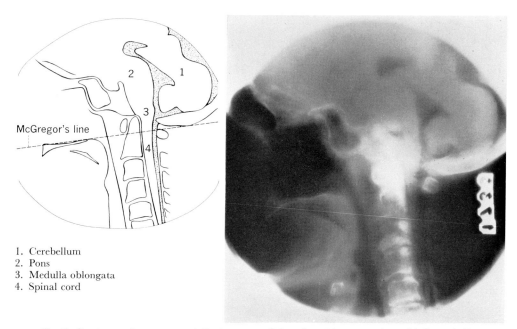

1. Cerebellum
2. Pons
3. Medulla oblongata
4. Spinal cord

C. Basilar impression — upward displacement of the odontoid process above McGregor's line and relative descending of the medulla oblongata below the foramen magnum.

Fig. 107 (A–C) Pneumoencephalography. (Courtesy of Dr. N. KOBAYASHI)

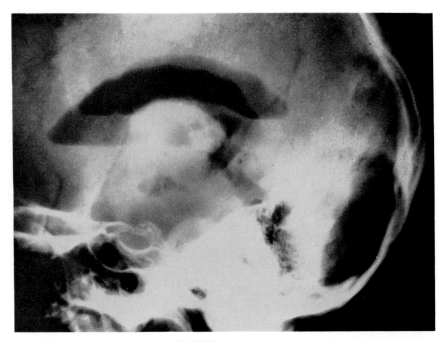

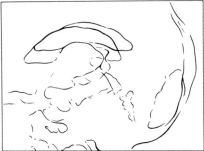

A. Lateral view: enlargement of the lateral ventricle and atrophy of the cerebellum is observed.

Fig. 108 Controlled pneumoencephalography.

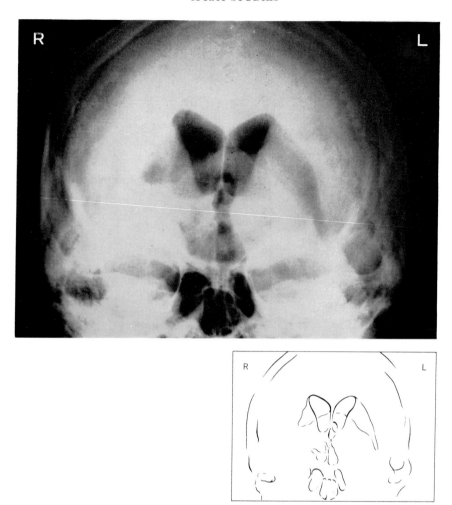

B. Frontal view: enlargement of the lateral ventricle is observed.

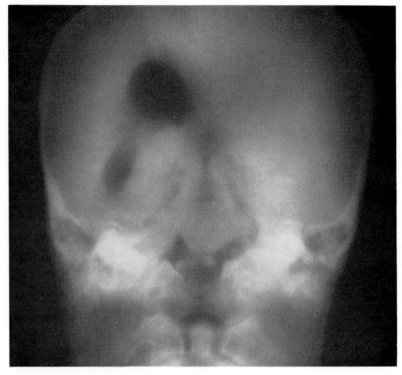

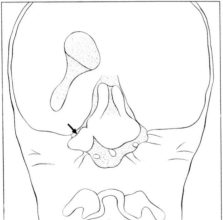

Fig. 109 Combined PEG and circus tomography.

A mass at the left cerebellopontine angle is clearly outlined by the gas shadow (arrow).
The eroded internal auditory canal is also shown.

IV

The Interpretation of Test Results

PERIPHERAL VERSUS CENTRAL VESTIBULAR DISTURBANCES

Although mention has been made of a host of diagnostic tests and procedures in the preceding chapters, the readers will not infrequently encounter difficulty in solving diagnostic problems. The first step in determining a correct diagnosis should be to decide the location of pathology. One may find assistance in the following list of findings which help to distinguish between peripheral and central vestibular disturbances.

The findings listed can be regarded as strongly indicative of either peripheral or central lesion. Nevertheless, these findings should be correlated with other evidence before drawing a conclusion.

1. Signs and Symptoms Indicative of a Peripheral Lesion
a. Recurrent attacks of vertigo accompanying cochlear symptoms
b. Transitory rotatory nystagmus together with vertigo on the positioning nystagmus test, which is lessened by successive repetition of the test or changes direction with return to the sitting position—Gegenläufigkeit.
c. Presence of hypo- or non-excitability of the vestibular labyrinth clearly demonstrated by the caloric test.
d. Presence of vestibular recruitment indicated by self-recording cupulometry.
e. Occurrence of nystagmus by the pneumatic test for a labyrinthine fistula.

2. Signs and Symptoms Indicative of a Central Lesion
a. Vertigo and dizziness accompanying loss of consciousness or manifestation of involvement of the cranial nerves (other than the vestibulocochlear nerves), the long tracts or the cerebellum.
b. Gradually increasing disturbance of standing and walking without falling tendency to a certain direction.
c. Falling of the body in the direction of the quick phase of spontaneous nystagmus.
d. Non-episodic and persistent nystagmus, spontaneous or positional, without accompanying vertigo or cochlear symptoms.
e. Gross spontaneous vertical or diagonal nystagmus.
f. Spontaneous nystagmus with a dissociated nature.
g. Nystagmus directed bilaterally on non-extreme lateral gaze—gaze-direction nystagmus.
h. Coarse direction-changing positional nystagmus.
i. Vertical nystagmus with large amplitude on the positioning nystagmus test, which is reproducible by successive repetition of the test.
j. Perversion of caloric response.
k. Absence of vestibular recrutiment on the self-recording cupulometry.
l. Marked alteration of the optokinetic response.
m. Atactic eye movements in the eye-tracking test.
n. Absence of the quick phase of experimentally induced nystagmus.

V

Case Studies

1. MÉNIÈRE'S DISEASE

A 35 year-old housewife was in good health until three years previous when she began to experience attacks of vertigo. The vertiginous attacks were infrequent in the beginning, one attack during several months; recently attacks became more frequent, several attacks occurring per month. The attacks were accompanied by vomiting and by cochlear signs, tinnitus, sensation of ear obstruction and difficulty in hearing on the right side.

Examination. Mental status, motor and sensory examination, and examination of coordination were unremarkable. Cranial nerves: other than the neuro-otological findings noted below, the cranial nerves were unremarkable.

1) A low tone deafness of varying threshold with a positive recruitment phenomenon was demonstrated. Figs. 110 a,b show the air conduction threshold measured and nystagmus findings on two days during (V/2) and between attacks (V/16).

2) There was no gaze nystagmus. Positional and positioning nystagmus, horizontal-rotating and direction-fixed to the right was demonstrated during an attack and persisted for two weeks. The nystagmus was most pronounced during mental calculation (Fig. 111a,b). There was directionally different type or DP type of optokinetic pattern test (Fig. 111 c). Nystagmus beats directed to the right were superimposed on the eye tracking record (Fig. 112). Nothing abnormal was found on laboratory or X-ray examination.

This case is illustrative of a rather typical case of Ménière's disease.

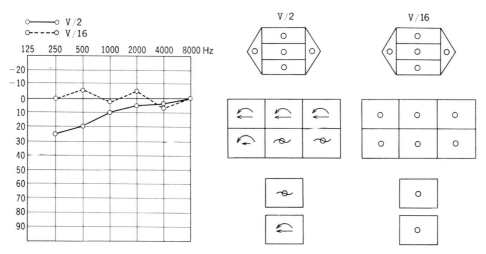

Fig. 110 a A threshold change in air conduction on the right.

Fig. 110 b Gaze, positional and positioning nystagmus findings.

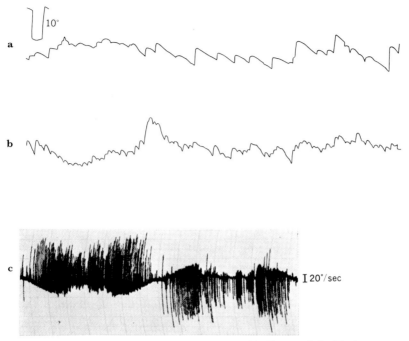

Fig. 111 Spontaneous nystagmus electronystagmographically recorded with the eyes covered (a) and with the eyes closed (b).   OKPs showed a remarkable side difference, better on the right, and worse on the left.

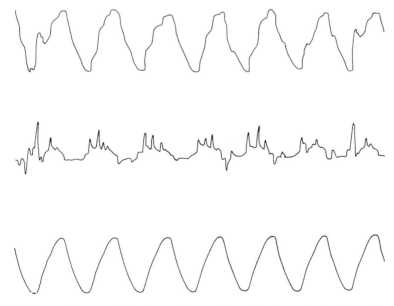

Fig. 112 Eye-tracking test induced saccades superimposed only on the tracking of the eyes toward the right.

(J. Suzuki)

2. LABYRINTHITIS SECONDARY TO CHOLESTEATOMA OTITIS

A 42 year-old male came to the hospital complaining of vertigo and otorrhea of the right ear.

The patient had a history of intermittent episodic recurrent discharge from the right ear since childhood, lasting usually for about a week. Two months before admission otorrhea appeared after having caught cold. While receiving local installation of antibiotic solution in the ear a turning sensation sometimes appeared, but subsided within a few minutes. From one day before admission, he felt a sensation of objects swaying from side to side. The vertigo was much exaggerated and accompanied by nausea, after treatment of the right ear. On the day of admission his vertigo was so severe that he could not raise his head.

Examination. His general medical examination was not remarkable. There was an attic perforation in the right tympanic membrane through which a cholesteatoma could be seen. No abnormalities of the left tympanic membrane were found. Audiometry showed a severe mixed-type hearing loss of the right ear. Although no spontaneous nystagmus was present in the sitting position, the positional and positioning tests revealed transitory nystagmus of varying type, i.e. horizontal nystagmus to the affected side, and downward or rotatory nystagmus (Fig. 113). The caloric test showed an active response with 20 °C stimulation of the left ear, but to stimulation of the right ear only a weak response could be elicited with 10 °C water. A fistula test appeared to be negative as compression of air in the external meatus did not produce vertigo or nystagmus.

Operation and postoperative course. At surgery a cholesteatoma which dipped into the antrum, aditus and epitympanum was found. As the cholesteatoma matrix was removed, the lateral semicircular canal was exposed for a length of about 3 mm. There was necrosis of the upper portions of the incus and malleus, but the stapes was intact. Type III tympanoplasty, producing a myringostapediopexy, was performed by using a fascia graft from the temporal muscle.

The postoperative course was uneventful. The positional and positioning tests done 5 days after surgery revealed horizontal nystagmus to the left in all head positions. The caloric test using 5 ml of Colimycin solution adjusted at 10 °C did not produce any reaction from the right ear. Five months later, spontaneous nystagmus to the left disappeared except during eye closure.

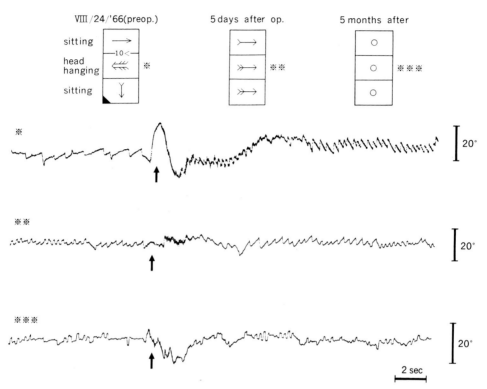

Fig. 113   The positioning tests from the sitting to the head-hanging position with the eyes open in darkness (time constant 1.5 seconds, bitemporal leads).

(T. Uemura)

3. VESTIBULAR NEURONITIS

A 19 year-old male was well until about 20 days prior to seeking medical attention when he caught cold and noticed posterior nasal discharge and cough.   Two weeks later he noted a turning sensation when he suddenly turned his head to the left, but neither tinnitus nor deafness was noticed.   This vertigo lasted for a few days and then changed to a swaying sensation of his entire body.

On examination his general condition was good and he was able to walk without support. The mucous membrane of the nose and pharynx was slightly inflamed. Otherwise there were no remarkable findings in the ear, nose or throat.   Horizontal-rotatory nystagmus to the right was observed on lateral gaze to the right.   The corneal reflex was normal.   Neither facial nor soft palate involvement was present.   Hearing in both ears was normal.

Results of the equilibrium function test showed that he was able to stand on one leg with eyes open, but was not able to stand on one leg with his eyes closed.   The vertical writing test revealed a deviation to the left.   The ENG showed horizontal nystagmus to the right, its magnitude decreasing progressively when the eyes were closed, open in darkness, and with Frenzel glasses.   No nystagmus was recorded under the visual fixation condition (Fig. 114; I/28/'66).   The intensity of nystagmus decreased in the right side down position and increased in the left side down position, i.e. it was direction-fixed positional nystagmus. The caloric test was performed using 20 °C water and nystagmus was recorded by ENG with the eyes open in darkness.   Changes in the intensity of nystagmus after irrigation are presented on the graph by plotting the values of the slow phase speed measured at 15 sec intervals (Fig. 115).   The lack of appearance of nystagmus after right ear stimulation does not imply a lack of caloric response, as spontaneous nystagmus was beating to the opposite side.   However, it is not clear whether the slight exacerbation of nystagmus intensity after left ear stimulation (Fig. 115 a) is calorically induced nystagmus or can be explained by exacerbation of spontaneous nystagmus secondary to a general alerting reaction.   To address this question stronger stimulation with 10 °C water was applied.   Although the right-sided stimulation produced nystagmus to the left as might be expected (Fig. 115 b), left-sided stimulation caused only the exacerbation of spontaneous nystagmus to the same extent as in the 20 °C stimulation.   This result thus indicates the existence of severe or complete canal paresis of the left side.

Laboratory test: White cell count was 12,000/cu mm and differential count was normal.   The serologic examination for syphilis was negative.   Other laboratory tests and X-ray examination were normal.

Course. An ENG 20 days after admission revealed spontaneous nystagmus only when the eyes were closed (Fig. 114, lower traces).   The caloric test revealed a clear but weak response from the left ear (Fig. 115 c).   This case was diagnosed as vestibular neuronitis.

Comments. Vestibular neuronitis has characteristic features, according to Dix and Hallpike (1952), as follows: A chief complaint of vertigo not accompanied by cochlear symptoms; spontaneous nystagmus to the intact side; a reduction of the caloric and galvanic responses on the affected side and acute infection of the upper respiratory tract preceding the onset of the illness.   It is still questionable whether this complex can be differentiated from other peripheral labyrinthine diseases or cranial mononeuritis as a separate disease entity.

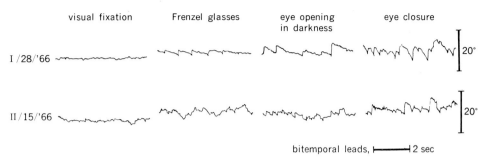

Fig. 114 The spontaneous nystagmus tests.

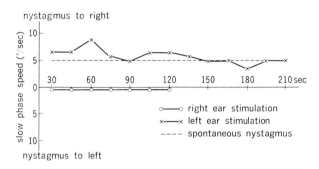

a. 20 °C stimulation (I/28/'66)

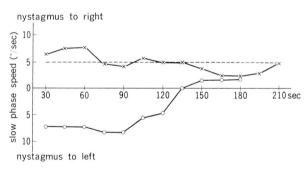

b. 10 °C stimulation (I/28/'66)

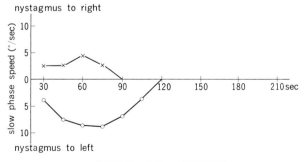

c. 20 °C stimulation (II/15/'66)

Fig. 115 Results of the caloric tests.

(T. UEMURA)

4. SUDDEN DEAFNESS

A 21 year-old businessman was admitted to the hospital complaining of sudden right-sided hearing loss and dizziness. Five days prior to admission, when he got up in the morning, he noted nausea, hearing loss, and tinnitus in his right ear. Later that afternoon, he felt that the room started to turn clockwise and his nausea became more severe.

On examination his general condition was good and he was able to walk without help. The otoscopic examination was not remarkable. Spontaneous nystagmus was not observed in the sitting position. The corneal reflex was normal. Neither facial nor soft palate palsy was present. His blood pressure was 120/70.

The hearing test: An audiogram showed severe sensorineural hearing loss in the right ear (Fig. 116, XII/18). The hearing acuity of the left ear was normal.

The equilibrium function test: Although he was able to stand on one leg with open eyes, standing on one leg with closed eyes was impossible. The vertical writing test revealed a deviation to the left (Fig. 12 a, before treatment). ENG showed nystagmus to the left in the supine and left lateral positions and to the right in the right lateral position, i.e. divergent (or geotropic) direction-changing positional nystagmus (Fig. 117, top traces). The caloric test using 20 °C water revealed equally active responses in both ears. Laboratory tests, including serology and skull X-ray were unremarkable.

Course. Stellate ganglion block and medical treatment were begun. Four days after admission he noticed subjective improvement of his hearing and the audiograms tested successively showed a gradual recovery in the low and middle frequency ranges (Fig. 116, XII/22, XII/25). However, the hearing loss beyond 2,000 Hz remained almost unchanged for one year. The direction-changing positional nystagmus became converted to spontaneous nystagmus to the left 10 days after onset and further to the convergent (or apogeotropic) direction-changing type 24 days after onset (Fig. 117, middle and bottom traces).

Comments. Since the clinical features of sudden deafness are different from those in the typical case of Ménière's disease, it appears to be reasonable that both should be considered separately until their underlying causes are clarified.

125
250
500
1000
2000
4000
8000 Hz
-30
-20
-10
0
10
20
30
40
50
60
70
80
90
100
dB
XII/25
XII/22
XII/18
800
1500
3000
6000
10000

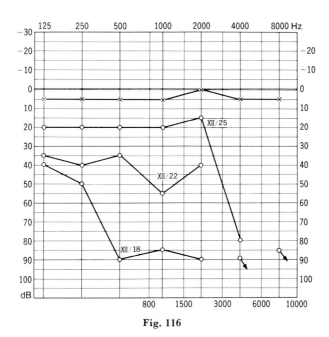

Fig. 116

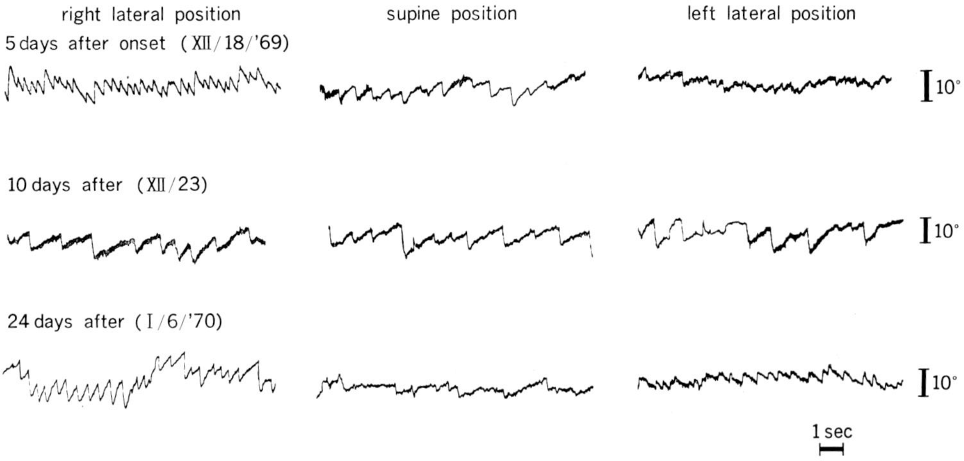

right lateral position
supine position
left lateral position
5 days after onset (XII/18/'69)
10°
10 days after (XII/23)
10°
24 days after (I/6/'70)
10°
1 sec

Fig. 117 The positional tests (eye opening in darkness, bitemporal leads).

(T. Uemura)

5. CERVICOVESTIBULAR SYNDROME

A 50 year-old man was well until six months previous to admission to the hospital.   At that time the patient noticed that episodes of vertigo were provoked particularly by turning his head to the left side.   He also complained of left sided tinnitus, but hearing loss was not noticed.   These attacks would continue for several seconds or minutes without unconsciousness.

On examination the mental status was non-remarkable.   The neuro-otologic examination revealed a characteristic HORNER's syndrome was on the left and left VIIIth nerve dysfunction as listed below.

Findings of nystagmus tests rotatory nystagmus provoked by the positioning test.   This nystagmus was accompanied by vertigo, and showed so-called "Gegenlaüfigkeit" (STENGER, 1955).   By repeating the test "fatigue of nystagmus" (LINDSAY, 1951) was characteristic.   This nystagmus was thought to originate from a peripheral vestibular disturbance.

X-ray examination of the spine showed spondylosis deformans $C_{5,6}$.   Arteriograms revealed "kinking" near the proximal portion of the left vertebral artery.   This was manifested when the neck was turned to the left (Fig. 118).

Otologic findings: Organic disease of the ear was not found by otoscopic and X-ray examinations.   Hearing was normal in both ears.

Diagnosis and treatment.   This patient was diagnosed to be a case of the peripheral type of cervicovestibular syndrome.   Perivascular sympathectomy was carried out at the proximal portion of the left vertebral artery.   After the operation, the episodes of vertigo and positioning nystagmus disappeared.   The abnormal findings of the cupulometric examination also disappeared (Fig. 119).

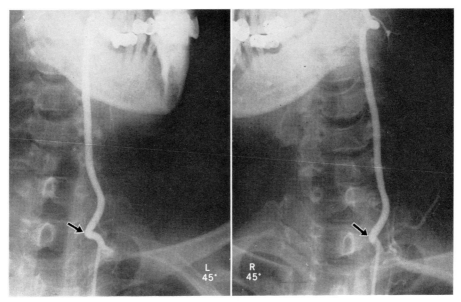

Fig. 118 Vertebral angiography.
"Kinking" can be observed near the proximal portion of the left vertebral artery which was manifested when the neck was turned to the left.

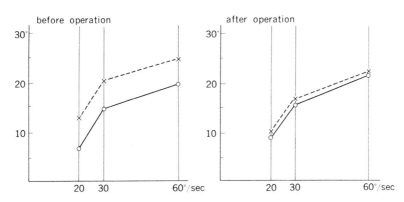

Fig. 119 Cupulometric findings before and after operation.
This case showed the parallel type cupulogram before the operation. But the width between the two lines decreased in accordance with improvement of vertigo after the operation.
○——○ clockwise rotation   × . . . . × counter-clockwise rotation

(J. HOZAWA)

6. ACOUSTIC NEURINOMA

A 38 year-old man who complained of disturbed equilibrium and left-sided hearing loss was admitted to the hospital.

Ten months prior to admission, the patient noticed difficulty in keeping his balance while skiing. He also noted clumsiness when standing on one leg with his eyes closed. Left-sided hearing loss and hypoesthesia of the left side of the lips and cheek were noted at the same time. Occipital and frontal headaches were present for two months prior to admission. On admission, although he sometimes felt nausea, there was no vomiting, vertigo, or tinnitus.

General medical examination was unremarkable. Visual acuity, visual field and pupillary reflex were normal. Appearance of the optic disc was normal. The left corneal reflex was depressed. Coarse gaze nystagmus to the left was present on left lateral gaze (Fig. 120 a). Incomplete peripheral facial paralysis was noted on the left side, but there was no gaze palsy or soft palate palsy. Coordination of hand movements was slightly impaired on the left side.

The hearing test (Fig. 121): The right ear was normal, and there was a moderate sensorineural deafness with positive recruitment phenomenon* in the left ear.

The equilibrium function test: Standing on one or both legs with eyes open was normal; standing on one leg with eyes closed was grossly abnormal. The vertical writing test with the right hand did not indicate abnormality. Diagonal downward nystagmus with the horizontal component to the right was noted in the left side down position under Frenzel glasses and with the eyes open in darkness (Fig. 120 b, left). However, positional nystagmus to the left was recorded in the same position during eye closure (Fig. 120 b, right). The positioning test from the sitting to the head-hanging position revealed a combination of downward and left beating nystagmus, and reverse positioning to the sitting position revealed diagonal upward nystagmus. The caloric test using 20 °C water was normal in the right ear but no response was obtained from the left ear even with 10 °C stimulation.

X-ray films of the petrous pyramid demonstrated an enlargement of the left internal auditory canal. The lumbar puncture was clear and colorless; 130 mmH$_2$O; cell count 1/3; Pandy (╫); protein 107 mg/dl; Queckenstedt (−). Diagnosis of acoustic neurinoma was made.

Operation and postoperative course. Through occipital craniotomy a $3 \times 2 \times 2$ cm acoustic neurinoma was completely removed. Although the patient was relieved of nausea and facial hypoesthesia, he lost all hearing in the left ear and his left facial nerve function was permanently lost.

Comments. It is apparent that this patient will remain disabled, even though the tumor was successfully removed. The importance of diagnosis of acoustic neurinoma at the "ear tumor" or early stage must be emphasized since the treatment becomes progressively more difficult and the prognosis worsens as the tumor enlarges. When progressive unilateral hearing loss is present, acoustic neurinoma must therefore be suspected.

---

* The presence of recruitment phenomenon in cases of acoustic neurinoma is rather rare, and it may be explained by a concomitant cochlear damage due to involvement of cochlear blood supply by tumor pressure.

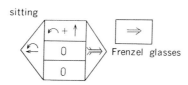

Fig. 120 a   Spontaneous nystagmus.

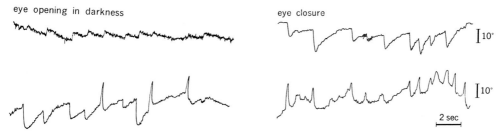

Fig. 120 b   Positional nystagmus in the left lateral position.
In each pair the upper trace was obtained with a 1.5 second time constant through the bitemporal
leads and the lower trace through the vertical leads.

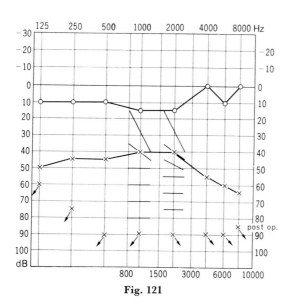

Fig. 121

(T. UEMURA)

7. ACOUSTIC NEURINOMA (GIANT TUMOR TYPE)

A 36 year-old housewife was well until five months previous to admission when she noticed pains on the left side of the head, face and inside of the mouth. She also complained of dizziness, staggering to the left, left sided tinnitus and hearing loss. Two months before admission she noticed worsening of the above complaints as well as the new complaints of sagging of the left side of the face and difficulty with speech. One month before admission, she noticed double vision on leftward gaze, pain around the left eye and morning dizziness.

On examination the mental status was non-remarkable. The cranial nerves examination showed bilateral low grade choked disc, diminished left sided facial sensation including an absent left corneal reflex, left lateral rectus palsy, left facial palsy (peripheral type including impairment of taste), left sided deafness and absent caloric response on the left side.

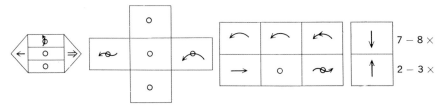

Fig. 122 Spontaneous and positional nystagmus tests.

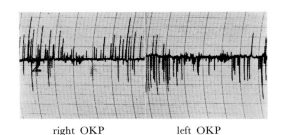

right OKP   left OKP

Fig. 123   OKP test.

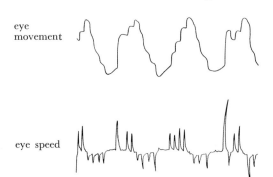

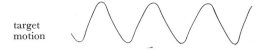

Fig. 124 Eye tracking test.

On examination of the motor system muscle strength was undiminished, but coordination was impaired on the left, deep tendon-reflexes were 3+ bilaterally.

The sensory examination was unremarkalbe.

Equilibrium function tests: ROMBERG's test was positive. Bilateral course gaze nystagmus (BRUNS' type), positive positional and positioning nystagmus of the direction-changing type were noted. In addition, vertical positioning nystagmus in the sagittal plane was revealed. OKP test was highly defective and showed little side difference. Eye tracking was abnormal of the stair-step type and was partially attactic.

Comments on neuro-otological examination. All of the neuro-otological findings indicated an extensive lesion in the infratentorial space: bilateral gaze nystagmus of BRUNS' type*, direction changing positional nystagmus, direction changing vertical positioning nystagmus, markedly defective OKP, coarse stair-step and partially atactic type of eye tracking, etc. Direction changing vertical positional nystagmus, which is common with spinocerebellar degeneration may indicate a lesion in the system, which inhibits nystagmus probably due to the interruption of cerebellar fibers.

(J. SUZUKI)

---

* **Fig. 125** BRUNS' nystagmus.

An example of a DC recording of the eye movements obtained from a patient with a right sided acoustic neurinoma in the "brain tumor" stage (upper traces). The record began from the position of direct forward gaze and the patient was instructed to look to the right and left in 10° steps. The room lights were on. Note that the nystagmus increased as the eyes deviated more laterally. The nystagmus on 30° gaze to the right was of large amplitude, while the nystagmus on 30° gaze to the left was of smaller amplitude and higher frequency. The lower traces are the differentiated ENG. The calibration for this trace is 50°/sec. (From Dr. UEMURA)

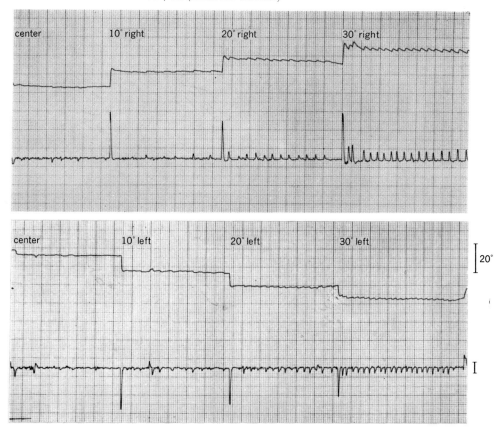

8. BRAINSTEM LESION DUE TO VERTEBRAL-BASILAR
INSUFFICIENCY

A 49 year-old man came to the hospital with the chief complaint of vertigo, hearing loss and facial weakness on the right side.   Over the past three years the patient was treated for hypertension (180/105 mmHg).   One month prior to admission, on arising he felt a severe turning sensation of his entire body associated with nausea and vomiting.   The vertigo continued for one week.   He also noted total deafness and tinnitus in his right ear as well as facial weakness of the right side.   However, there was no impairment of consciousness.

The neurological examination revealed hypoesthesia of the right side of the face, diminished right corneal reflex, and right peripheral facial paralysis.   There was no gaze palsy, soft palate, sensory or motor paralysis.   Funduscopic examination revealed no papilledema, but severe arteriosclerotic changes were noted.

The hearing test showed a profound hearing loss on the right and a high-tone hearing loss on the left (Fig. 126).

Equilibrium function tests showed that the patient could stand on one leg with eyes open but could not stand on one leg with his eyes closed.   Asymmetric bilateral gaze nystagmus, i.e. more frequent and smaller amplitude to the right and less frequent and larger amplitude to the left, as well as horizontal nystagmus to the left on straight forward gaze was present (Fig. 127).   This nystagmus changed to square waves toward the right under Frenzel glasses and with eyes open in darkness (Fig. 30d, p. 58).   The nystagmus was reversed to a horizontal nystagmus toward the right with eyes closed.   The difference in velocity between the quick and slow phases of this nystagmus was relatively small (Fig. 30d).   The caloric test using 20°C water was normal in the left ear, but there was no response in the right ear even with 10°C stimulation.

Blood pressure: right, 142/92; left, 140/88 mmHg.   Blood Wassermann reaction was negative.

Course.   The patient showed a slow but gradual improvement of his hearing loss and facial paralysis during the seven weeks of his admission.   Bilateral gaze nystagmus and horizontal nystagmus to the left on straight forward gaze also decreased or disappeared after seven weeks (Fig. 127, X/27/'65).

Comments.   The neuro-otological findings in this case were indicative of a cerebellopontine angle lesion, but the presence of a tumor was excluded by the course of the illness.

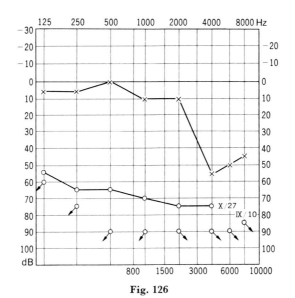

Fig. 126

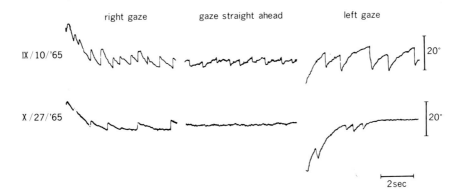

Fig. 127 Spontaneous nystagmus on ENG (time constant 1.5 sec, bitemporal leads).

(T. UEMURA)

9. WALLENBERG SYNDROME

A 43 year-old male clerk was well until about a month ago when he noticed decreased power of mastication on the right side.   The next day, a moderate discoordination of the limbs appeared, he could, however, still walk.   A week later, nausea with vomiting was noted and a dizzy sensation appeared for the first time.   Tongue movements became difficult.   Two days later nausea with vomiting worsened, walking without assistance was difficult, and double vision began.   No unconsciousness throughout the above course was reported.   He was hospitalized two weeks after the onset of symptoms.

Upon examination the mental status was normal.   The cranial nerve examination showed right-sided findings of blepharoptosis, HORNER's syndrome, abolished corneal reflex, weak mastication, abducens palsy, facial palsy, impaired taste, and a hemiparetic tongue.   The pharynx and larynx appeared normal.   Hearing and calorimetry were normal.   Rapidly alternating movements and coordination were impaired.   There were sensory deficits on the left side of the trunk and extremities.

Special tests including equilibrium function tests showed a positive ROMBERG.   Stepping with the eyes covered was grossly defective.   These was bilateral gaze nystagmus, and see-saw nystagmus with and without FRENZEL glasses.   Positional effects on the see-saw nystagmus were noted.   Vertical direction changing positioning nystagmus was also present as was a markedly impaired OKP.

Comments.   The case which may be included in the category of WALLENBERG syndrome is noted because of see-saw nystagmus.   In addition to this, the present case had several remarkable nystagmus findings: Bilateral gaze nystagmus indicating a pontine angle lesion; among other conditions, direction changing vertical positioning nystagmus strongly suggesting cerebellar involvements; an impaired OKP indicating an impaired optokinetic mechanism.   OKPs taken in the recovering course showed an improvement (Fig. 128).

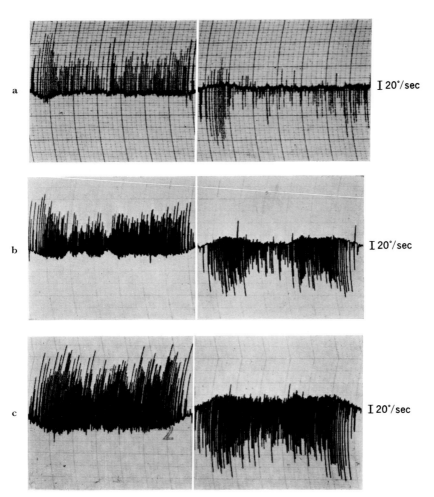

Fig. 128 Recovery of OKP depression on the 34th (a), 67th (b), and 104th (c) days
after the attack.

(J. Suzuki)

10. SUSPECTED BRAINSTEM AND CEREBELLUM LESION

This 20 year-old female secretary is now recovering from episodes of vertigo and staggering gait. About three years ago, she visited our vertigo clinic several times with the chief complaint of transient vertigo and a slightly staggering gait. Examination showed no neurological findings except for nystagmus: Gaze nystagmus with a strong clockwise rotation, geotropic direction-changing positional nystagmus and markedly rotating positioning nystagmus (Fig. 129 a). The OKP test was abnormal suggesting a possible lesion in the brainstem or cerebellum.

One year ago, she was hospitalized with a presumed diagnosis of tuberculous meningitis. She complained of severe headache and fever of a moderate degree. The spinal fluid was polycythemic or 326/3, with lymphoid cells. Cultures were negative including those for tuberclosis. Meningeal signs were equivocal. No other neurological signs were demonstrated except for neuro-otological findings: Marked non-gaze nystagmus mainly directing downward, direction changing type of positional nystagmus, coarse downward vertical positioning nystagmus (Fig. 129 b) were noted. The patient was begun on antituberculous medication.

About half a year ago, the above meningitis subsided. The complaints, presumably secondary to antituberculosis therapy at that time were of a slight dizzy sensation when she shook her head and of infrequent nausea. Nystagmus examination revealed some improvement at that time (Fig. 129 c).

The OKP test was markedly impaired throughout the three years course. Eye tracking was abnormal and of the fine stair-stepping type. Her writing was not disturbed and gait disturbance was not marked.

Comments. Most of the objective findings in this case were concentrated in the oculomotor system. These findings showed considerable variation during the three years course, but the main defects were two: 1) a defective inhibitory system which was indicated by geotropic positional nystagmus, and vertical positioning nystagmus, and 2) defective target following as revealed by both impaired optokinetic pattern and eye-tracking tests.

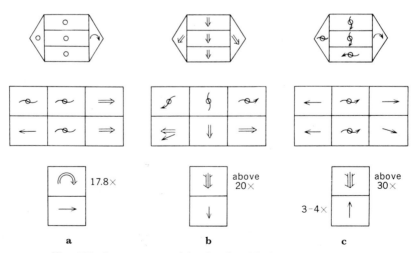

Fig. 129 Spontaneous, positional and positioning nystagmus tests.

(J. Suzuki)

11. CEREBELLAR ATAXIA

A 49 year-old male clerk complained of disturbed gait and speech. Speech disturbance appeared about a year ago with a relatively abrupt onset. Six months later, walking became gradually more difficult. There were no other complaints.

The examination showed that the mental status and cranial nerves were normal. The sensory examination was within normal limits, but the motor examination showed that coordination was markedly impaired. The patient had difficulty in standing on one foot, an atactic gait and dysdiadokokinesis. His hand writing was slightly impaired.

Standing unassisted was difficult. There was no gaze nystagmus and no positional nystagmus but coarse infrequent vertical positioning nystagmus directing downward was noted. There was an impaird OKP and a fine stair-stepped eye tracking response.

Comments. Nystagmus findings indicate no lateralization of the lesion. The coordination deficit, the positive findings with vertical positioning nystagmus, OKP and eye-tracking tests indicated some involvement of the oculomotor as well as the coordination mechanism. The lesion was most likely in the cerebellar midline.

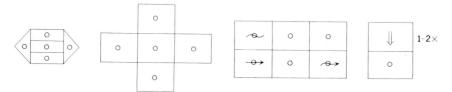

Fig. 130 Spontaneous and positional nystagmus tests.

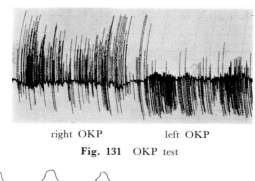

right OKP   left OKP

Fig. 131 OKP test

eye movement

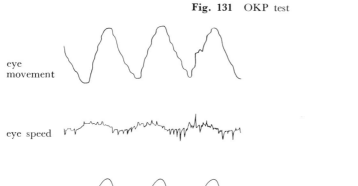

eye speed

target motion

Fig. 132 Eye-tracking test.

(J. SUZUKI)

12–1. PAROXYSMAL POSITIONING VERTIGO

A 35 year-old housewife complained of episodic vertigo. During the past 5 years, once a year or so, she suffered from episodes of vertigo accompanied by nausea lasting for several days. No tinnitus, nor hearing loss was noted. Head movements induced a vertiginous sensation. No other neurological complaints were present.

Examination. Marked rotating positioning nystagmus which was direction-changing (Fig. 133) was noted. Other examinations of equilibrium were normal. There were no neurologic or positive laboratory findings.

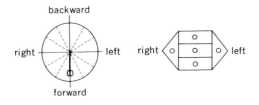

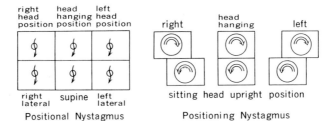

Fig. 133 Stepping test, and spontaneous, positional and positioning nystagmus tests.

(J. Suzuki)

12–2. PAROXYSMAL POSITIONAL VERTIGO

An 18 year-old female student complained of episodic vertigo.

The attacks of episodic positional vertigo occurred at varying intervals and were frequently accompanied by head colds. The right side down head position usually induced vertigo, but there was no tinnitus, deafness, or associated nausea. Torticollis to the left was noted.

Upon examination no psychiatric, or neurological findings were noted except for nystagmus induced by head position changes. Tilting the head to the right usually provoked vertigo. As shown in Fig. 134, strong nystagmus was observed in the several head positions which were tested. The nystagmus was horizontal rotating or rotating, and the direction was sometimes reversed. Head position change against gravity modified the nystagmus but merely twisting the neck was not effective. Calorization was not responsive on the left side.

Comments. The above two cases are similar in having no neurological findings except for the nystagmus induced by head position changes. Head positioning was effective in Case 12–1, while only particular head positions without positioning effect were noted in the Case 12–2. Most of episodic positional or positioning vertigo cases are benign and have no neurological findings including hearing and caloric functions. Cases similar to these appear to be more frequent than Ménière's disease.

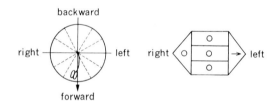

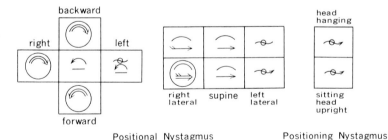

Fig. 134 Stepping test, and spontaneous, positional and positioning nystagmus tests.

(J. Suzuki)

Bibliography

AANTAA, E. (1970): Light-induced and spontaneous variations in amplitude of the electro-oculogram. Acta oto-laryng., Suppl. 267.

ADAMS, A. (1957): Nystagmographische Untersuchungen über den Lidnystagmus und die physiologische Koordination von Lidschlag und rascher Nystagmusphase. Arch. Ohr.-, Nas.-, u. Kehlk.-Heilk., *170*: 543–558.

ADAMS, A. und STAEWEN, CH. (1959): Das Electronystagmogramm (ENG) bei Krankheiten des Zentralnervensystem und Hirntraumen. Dtsch. Z. Nervenheilk., *178*: 614–638.

ALFARO, V. R. (1958): Diagnostic significance of fulness in the ear. J.A.M.A., *166*: 239–245.

ALPERS, B. J. and YASKIN, H. E. (1944): The Bruns syndrome. J. Nerv. & Ment. Dis., *100*: 115–134.

ALPERS, B. J. (1958): Vertigo and Dizziness. Grune and Stratton, New York.

ALTMANN, F. (1955): Entzündliche und degenerative Erkrankungen des peripheren Cochlear- und Vestibular-neurons. Fortschr. Hals-Nas.-Ohrenheik., *2*: 80–145, S. Karger, Basel-New York.

ANDERSEN, H. C. (1954): Directional preponderance in some intracranial disorders. Acta oto-laryng., *44*: 568–573.

ANDERSEN, H. C., JEPSEN, O. and KRISTIANSEN, F. (1954): The occurrence of directional preponderance in some intracranial disorders. Acta oto-laryng., Suppl. *118*: 19–31.

ARSLAN, M. (1953): Über die Methodik der Vestibularisuntersuchungen mit einem Vorschlag zur Standardisierung. Fortschr. Hals-Nas.-Ohrenheilk., *1*: 148–165, S. Karger, Basel-New York.

ARSLAN, M. (1955): On the renewing of the methodology for the stimulation of the vestibular apparatus. A discussion with clinical aims. Acta oto-laryng., Suppl. 122.

ASCHAN, G. (1955): The caloric test. A nystagmographical study. Acta Soc. Med. Upsal., *60*: 99–112.

ASCHAN, G. (1958): Cine nystagmography. Acta oto-laryng., *140*: 281–283.

ASCHAN, G. (1964): Nystagmography and caloric test. In: Neurological Aspects of Auditory and Vestibular Disorders (W.S. FIELDS and B.R. ALFORD eds.), pp. 216–247, C. C Thomas, Springfield, Ill.

ASCHAN, G. and BERGSTEDT, M. (1955): Non-vestibular nystagmus—a nystagmographic investigation. Acta Soc. Med. Upsal., *60*: 1–13.

ASCHAN, G., BERGSTEDT, M. and STAHLE, J. (1956): Nystagmography. Recording of nystagmus in clinical neuro-otological examinations. Acta oto-laryng., Suppl. 129.

Aschan, G. and STAHLE, J. (1956): Vestibular neuritis. A nystagmographical study. J. Laryng., *70*: 497–511.

ASCHAN, G., BERGSTEDT, M., NYLÉN, C.O. and STAHLE, J. (1957): The effect of head-movement on positional nystagmus—electronystagmography with an electric driven posture-table. Laryngoscope, *67*: 884–893.

ATKINS, A. and BENDER, M. B. (1964): Lightning eye movements (Ocular myoclonus). J. Neurol. Sci., *1*: 2–12.

ATKINSON, M. (1939): A simple quantitative method of testing vestibular function. Arch. Otolaryng., *30*: 916–921.

AZZI, A., GIORDANO, R. and SPELTA, O. (1953): Does a vestibular recruitment exist? Acta oto-laryng., *43*: 352–368.

BADER, W. und KORNHUBER, H. H. (1965): Grosshirnläsionen und vestibulärer Nystagmus. Vergleichende elektronystagmographische Untersuchungen bei geschlossenen Augen und mit visueller Fixation. Acta oto-laryng., *60*: 197–206.

BÁRÁNY, R. (1906): Über die vom Ohrlabyrinth ausglöste Gegenrollung der Augen bei Normalhörenden, Ohrenkrankheiten und Taubstummen. Arch. Ohrenheilk., *68*: 1–30.

BÁRÁNY, R. (1906): Untersuchungen über den vom Vestibularapparat des Ohres reflektorisch ausgelösten rhythmischen Nystagmus und seine Begleiterscheinungen. Mschr. Ohrenheilk., *40*: 193–297.

Bárány, R. (1907): Physiologie und Pathologie des Bogengangapparates beim Menschen. Veinna, Deuticke.

Bárány, R. (1911): Experimentelle Alkoholintoxikation. Mschr. Ohrenheilk., *45:* 959–961.

Bárány, R. (1911): Beziehungen zwischen Vestibularapparat und Cerebellum. Mschr. Ohrenheilk., *45:* 505–513.

Bárány, R. (1913): Dauernde Veränderung des spontanen Nystagmus bei Veränderung der Kopflage. Mschr. Ohrenheilk., *47:* 481–483.

Bárány, R. (1920): Zur Klinik und Theorie des Eisenbahnnystagmus. Acta oto-laryng., *3:* 260–265.

Bárány, R. (1921): Diagnose von Krankheitserscheinungen im Bereiche des Otolithenapparates. Acta oto-laryng., *2:* 434–437.

Békésy, G., von (1947): A new audiometer. Acta otolaryng., *35:* 411.

Bender, M. B. (1955): The eye-centering system. Arch. Neurol. Psychiat., *73:* 685–699.

Bender, M. B. (1960): Comments on the physiology and pathology of eye movements in the vertical plane. J. Nerv. Ment. Dis., *130:* 456–466.

Bender, M. B. (1965): Oscillopsia. Arch. Neurol., *13:* 204–213.

Bender, M.B. (ed.) (1967): The Approach to Diagnosis in Modern Neurology. Grune & Stratton, New York.

Bender, M. B. and Shanzer, S. (1964): Oculomotor pathways defined by electric stimulation and lesions in the brainstem of monkey. In: The Oculomotor System (M. B. Bender, ed.), pp. 81–140, Hoeber, New York.

Bender, M. B. and Weinstein, E. A. (1944): Effects of stimulation and lesion of the median longitudinal fasciculus in the monkey. Arch. Neurol. Psychiat., *52:* 106–113.

Benitez, J. T. (1970): Eye-tracking and optokinetic tests: diagnostic significance in peripheral and central vestibular disorders. Laryngoscope, *80:* 834–849.

Benjamin, C. E. (1926): Eine einfache Methode zur Messung der Gegenrollung des Auges. Arch. Ohr.-, Nas.-, u. Kehlk. Heilk. *115:* 210–215.

Bernstein, L. (1965): Simplification of clinical caloric test. Arch. Otolaryng., *81:* 347–349.

Black, F. O., Custer, D. D., Hemenway, W. G. and Thornby, J. I. (1973): The sequential bithermal binaural caloric test. II. clinical application of new statistical methods for interpretation. Ann. Otol., *82:* Suppl. *6:* 9–14.

Blomberg, L-H. (1959): The optokinetic fusion limit. Acta oto-laryng., *51:* 455–466.

Brain, W. R. (1938): Vertigo. Its neurological, otological, circulatory and surgical aspects. Brit. M. J., *2:* 605–608.

Brickner, R. M. (1936): Oscillopsia. A new symptom commonly occurring in multiple sclerosis. Arch. Neurol. Psychiat., *36:* 586–589.

Brodal, A. (1969): Neurological Anatomy. In Relation to Clinical Medicine. 2nd ed., Oxford University Press, New York.

Brodal, A., Pompeiano, O. and Walberg, F. (1962): The vestibular nuclei and their connections. Anatomy and functional correlations. The Henderson Trust Lectures. Oliver & Boyd, Edinburgh.

Brodman, K., Erdmann, A. J., Jr., Lorge, I. and Wolff, H. G. (1949): The Cornell medical index. An adjunct to medical interview. J.A.M.A., *140:* 530–534.

Brookler, K. H. (1971): Simultaneous bilateral bithermal caloric stimulation in electronystagmography. Laryngoscope, *81:* 1014–1019.

Bruner, A. and Norris, T. W. (1971): Age-related changes in caloric nystagmus. Acta oto-laryng. Suppl. 282.

Bruns (1902): Neuropathologische Demonstrationen. Neurol. Zbl., *21:* 561–567.

Buys (1909): Beitrag zum Studium des galvanischen Nystagmus mit Hilfe des Nystagmographen. Mschr. Ohrenheilk., *43:* 801–803.

Capps, M. J., Preciado, M. C., Pararella, M. M. and Hoppe, W. E. (1973): Evaluation of the air caloric test as a routine examination procedure. Laryngoscope, *83:* 1013–1021.

Carmichael, L. and Dearborn, W. F. (1947): Reading and Visual Fatigue. Houghton Mifflin Company, Boston. Quoted by Marg (1951).

Carmichael, E. A., Dix, M. R. and Hallpike, C. S. (1954): Lesions of the cerebral hemispheres and their effects upon optokinetic and caloric nystagmus. Brain, *77:* 345–372.

CARMICHAEL, E. A., DIX, M. R. and HALLPIKE, C. S. (1955): Disturbances of caloric and optokinetic nystagmus associated with localized lesions of the cerebral hemispheres. J. Laryng., *69:* 269–276.

CARMICHAEL, E. A., DIX, M. R., HALLPIKE, C. S. and HOOD, J. D. (1961): Some further observations upon the effect of unilateral cerebral lesions on caloric and rotational nystagmus. Brain, *84:* 571–584.

CAWTHORNE, T. E., FITZGERALD, G. and HALLPIKE, C. S. (1942): Studies in human vestibular function: II. Observations on the directional preponderance of caloric nystagmus ("Nystagmusbereitschaft") resulting from unilateral labyrinthectomy. Brain, *65:* 138–160.

CAWTHORNE, T. (1964): Otological aspects in the differential diagnosis of vertigo. In: Neurological aspects of auditory and vestibular disorders. (W.S. FIELDS and B.R. ALFORD eds.), pp. 271–282, C.C Thomas, Springfield, Ill.

CAWTHORNE, T. and COBB, W. A. (1954): Temperature changes in the perilymph space in response to caloric stimulation in man. Acta oto-laryng., *44:* 580–588.

CAWTHORNE, T. E., FITZGERALD, G. and HALLPIKE, C. S. (1942): Studies in human vestibular function: III. Observations on the clinical features of "Ménière's" disease with special reference to the results of the caloric tests. Brain, *65:* 161–180.

CAWTHORNE, T. and HINCHCLIFFE, R. (1961): Positional nystagmus of the central type as evidence of subtentorial metastases. Brain, *84:* 415–426.

COATS, A. C. (1966): Directional preponderance and spontaneous nystagmus. As observed in the electronystagmographic examination. Ann. Otol., *75:* 1135–1159.

COATS, A. C. (1968): Central and peripheral optokinetic asymmetry. Ann. Otol., *77:* 938–948.

COATS, A. C. (1969): Vestibular neuronitis. Acta oto-laryng. Suppl. 251.

COATS, A. C. (1970): Central electronystagmographic abnormalities. Arch. Otolaryng., *92:* 43–53.

COBURN, E. B. (1905): Arch. Ophthal. *34:* 1. Quoted by VERNON (1928).

COGAN, O. G. (1945): Syndrome of non-syphilitic interstitial keratitis and vestibuloauditory symptoms. Arch. Ophthal., *33:* 144–149.

COGAN, D. G. (1954): Ocular dysmetria; flutter-like oscillations of the eyes, and opsoclonus. Arch. Ophthal., *51:* 318–335.

COGAN, D. G. (1959): Convergence nystagmus. With notes on a single case of divergence nystagmus. Arch. Ophthal., *62:* 295–299.

COHEN, B. (1971): Vestibulo-ocular relations. In: The Control of Eye Movements (P. BACK-y-RITA and C.C. COLLINS eds.), pp. 105–148, Academic Press, New York-London.

COHEN, B., GOTO, K., SHANZER, S. and WEISS, A. H. (1965): Eye movements induced by electric stimulation of the cerebellum in the alert cat. Expr. Neurol., *13:* 145–162.

COHEN, B., GOTO, K. and TOKUMASU, K. (1967): Return eye movements, an ocular compensatory reflex in the alert cat and monkey. Expr. Neurol., *17:* 172–185.

COHEN, B., KOMATSUZAKI, A. and BENDER, M. B. (1968): Electro-oculographic syndrome in monkeys after pontine reticular formation lesions. Arch. Neurol., *18:* 78–92.

COHEN, B. and SUZUKI, J. (1963): Eye movements induced by ampullary nerve stimulation. Amer. J. Physiol., *204:* 347–351.

COHEN, B., SUZUKI, J. and BENDER, M. B. (1964): Eye movements from semicircular canal nerve stimulation in the cat. Ann. Otol., *73:* 153–169.

COHEN, B., SUZUKI, J. and BENDER, M. B. (1965): Nystagmus induced by semicircular canal nerve stimulation. Acta oto-laryng., *60:* 422–436.

COHEN, B., TOKUMASU, K. and GOTO, K. (1966): Semicircular canal nerve eye and head movements.—The effect of changes in initial eye and head position on the plane of the induced movement. Arch. Ophthal., *76:* 523–531.

COLLINS, W. E., GUEDRY, F. E., Jr. and POSNER, J. B. (1962): Control of caloric nystagmus by manipulating arousal and visual fixation distance. Ann. Otol., *71:* 187–202.

COPE, S. and RYAN, G.M.S. (1959): Cervical and otolith vertigo. J. Laryng., *73:* 113–120.

CORDS, R. (1927): Über Hebelnystagmographie. Graefes Arch. Ophthal., *118:* 771–784.

CORVEXA, J., TORRES-COURTNEY, G. and LOPEZ-RIONS, G. (1973): The neurotological significance of alterations of pursuit eye movements and the pendular eye tracking test. Ann. Otol., *82:* 855–867.

CUNNINGHAM, D. R. and BOETZINGER, C. P. (1972): Floor ataxia test battery. Results from an 8- to 18-year old group. Arch. Otolaryng., *96:* 559–564.

CUSTER, D. D., BLACK, F. O., HEMENWAY, W. G. and THORNBY, J. I. (1973): The sequential bithermal binaural caloric test. I. A statistical analysis of normal subject responses. Ann. Otol., *82:* Suppl. *6:* 3–8.

DAYAL, U. S., TARANTINO, L. and SWISHER, L. P. (1966): Neuro-otologic studies in multiple sclerosis. Laryngoscope, *76:* 1798–1809.

DE KLEIJN, A. and VERSTEEGH, C. (1924): Method of determining the compensatory positions of the human eye. Acta oto-laryng., *6:* 170–174.

DENNY-BROWN, D. (1953): Basilar artery syndromes. Bull. New England Med. Cent., *15:* 53–60.

DIX, M. R. and HALLPIKE, C. S. (1952): The pathology, symptomatology and diagnosis of certain common disorders of the vestibular system. Ann. Otol., *61:* 987–1026.

DIX, M.R. and HALLPIKE, C.S. (1960): Discussion on acoustic neuroma. Laryngoscope, *70:* 105–122.

DIX, M. R. and HALLPIKE, C. S. (1966): Observations on the clinical features and neurological mechanism of spontaneous nystagmus resulting from unilateral acoustic neurofibromata. Acta oto-laryng., *61:* 1–22.

DIX, M. R. and HOOD, J. D. (1970): Vestibular habituation, its clinical significance and relationship to vestibular neuronitis. Laryngoscope, *80:* 226–232.

DODGE, R. (1921): A mirror-recorder for photographing the compensatory movements of closed eyes. J. Exp. Psychol., *4:* 165–174.

DODGE, R. and CLINE, T. S. (1902): The angle velocity of eye movements. Psychol. Rev., *8:* 145–157. Quoted by VERNON (1928) and FERNANDEZ & LINDSAY (1965).

DOHLMAN, G. F. (1925): Physikalische und physiologische Studien zur Theorie des kalorischen Nystagmus. Acta oto-laryng., Suppl. 5.

DONDERS, F. C. (1890): Die Bewegungen des Auges, veranschaulich durch das Panophthalmotrop. Graefes Arch. Ophthal., *16:* 154–175.

du BOIS-REYMOND, E. (1949): Untersuchungen über thierische Electricität, Vol. 2-1, p. 256, G. Reimer, Berlin. Cited from MARG (1951).

DUENSING, F. and SCHAEFER, K. P. (1958): Die Aktivität einzelner Neurone im Bereich der Vestibularis Kerne bei Horizontal beschleunigung unter besonder Berücksichtigung des vestibulären Nystagmus. Arch. Psychiat. Nervenkr., *198:* 225–252.

DYKEN, P. and KOLÁŘ, O. (1968): Dancing eyes, dancing feet: infantile polymyoclonia. Brain, *91:* 305–320.

EDWARDS, C. H. and PATERSEN, J. H. (1951): A review of the symptoms and signs of acoustic neurofibromata. Brain, *74:* 144–190.

EGMOND, A. A. J., van und GROEN, G.G (1955): Cupulometrie. Pract. oto-rhino-laryng., *17:* 206–223.

EGMOND, A. A. J., van and JONGKEES, L.B.W. (1948): The turning test with small regulable stimuli. J. Laryng., *62:* 63–69.

ENGSTRÖM, H. (1958): On the double innervation of the sensory epithelia of the inner ear. Acta oto-laryng., *49:* 109–118.

EPISTEIN, B. (1950): The roentgenologic manifestation of acoustic neuroma. Amer. J. Roentgenol., *64:* 265–276.

EWALD, J. (1892): Physiologische Untersuchungen über das Endorgan des Nervus Octavus., Wiesbaden.

EVIATAR, A. (1970): The torsion swing as a vestibular test. Arch. Otolaryng., *92:* 437–444.

EVIATAR, A., GOODHILL, V. and WASSERTHEIL, S. (1970): The significance of spontaneous and positional nystagmus recorded by electronystagmography. As an independent test. Ann. Otol., *79:* 1117–1128.

FENN, W. O. and HURSH, J. B. (1937): Movements of the eyes when the lids are closed. Amer. J. Physiol., *118:* 8–14.

FERNANDEZ, C. and LINDSAY, J. R. (1965): Vestibular tests: methods of recording eye movements. Arch. Otolaryng., *82:* 664–666.

FIELDS, W. S. and WEIBEL, J. (1964): Effects of vascular disorders on the vestibular system. In: Neurological Aspects of Auditory and Vestibular Disorders (W. S. FIELDS and B.R. ALFORD eds.), pp. 305–335, C. C Thomas, Springfield, Ill.

FISCHER, J.J. (1956): The Labyrinth, Physiology and Functional Tests. Grune & Stratton, New York, London.

FISCHER, M. H. (1928): Die Regulationsfunktion des menschlichen Labyrinths. Bergmann, München.

FISCHER, M. H. (1930): Messende Untersuchungen über die Gegenrollung der Augen und die Lokalisation der scheinbaren bei seitlicher Neigung des Gesamtkörpers bis zu 360°: II Mitteilung. Untersuchung an Normalen. Graefes Arch. Ophthal., *123:* 476–508.

FISCHER, M. H. und WODAK, Z. (1923): Beiträge zur Physiologie des menschlichen Vestibular-apparates. I., II. Pflüg. Arch. Physiol., *202:* 522–552; 553–565.

FITZGERALD, G. and HALLPIKE, C. S. (1942): Studies in human vestibular function: I. Observations on the directional preponderance ("Nystagmusbereitschaft") of caloric nystagmus resulting from cerebral lesions. Brain, *65:* 115–137.

FLUUR, E. (1961): Efferent influences on vestibular functions following unilateral labyrinthectomy. Acta oto-laryng., *53:* 571–577.

FOWLER, E. P. (1936): A method for the early detections of otosclerosis. Arch. Otolaryng., *24:* 731–741.

FRENZEL, H. (1938 a): Das Fahnden nach Spontannystagmus, der wichtigste Vestibularisuntersuchung in der Praxis. Z. Hals-, u. Ohrenheilk., *44:* 347–358.

FRENZEL, H. (1938 b): Das Fahnden nach Spontannystagmus, der wichtigste Teil der Vestibularis-untersuchung in der Praxis. Z. Hals- Nas.- u. Ohrenheilk., *44:* 347–358.

FRENZEL, H. (1942): Hüpfender Nystagmus, eine besondere Schlagfrom des Spontannystagmus. Nervenarzt, *18:* 205–210.

FRENZEL, H. (1955): Spontan- u. Provokation-Nystagmus als Krankheitssymptom. Springer, Berlin, Göttingen, Heidelberg.

FRENZEL, H. (1957): Über den heutigen Stand der Funktionsprüfung des Vestibularis. II. Die moderne Entwicklung. Dtsch. med. Wschr., *82:* 372–378.

FRENZEL, H. (1959): Zur Frage einer Routinetechnik der thermischen Vestibularerregung. HNO, *7:* 353–358.

FRENZEL, H. (1961): Zur Systematik, Klinik und Untersuchungsmethodik der Vestibularisstö-rungen. Arch. Ohr.-, Nas.-, u. Kehlk.- Heilk., *177:* 353–395.

FRENZEL, H. und TONNDORF, E. EB. (1957): Zur Frage der Nystagmusmobilization infolge geschlossenen Augen und durch die Dunkelheit sowie zur Frage der Ausschaltung der Fixation durch die Leuchtbrille. Pract. oto-rhino-laryng., *19:* 507–517.

FUKAMACHI, K. (1959): The study on the Cornell Medical Index (I). Fukuoka Acta Med., *50:* 2988–3000. (in Japanese)

FUKAMACHI, K. (1959): The study on the Cornell Medical Index (II). Fukuoka Acta Med., *50:* 3001–3009. (in Japanese)

FUKUDA, T. (1959 a): Vertical writing with eyes covered. A new test of vestibulo-spinal reaction. Acta oto-laryng., *50:* 26–36.

FUKUDA, T. (1959 b): The stepping test. Two phases of the labyrinthine reflex. Acta oto-laryng., *50:* 95–108.

FUKUDA, T. (1961): Studies on human dynamic postures from the viewpoint of postural reflexes. Acta oto-laryng., Suppl. 161.

FUKUDA, T. and HINOKI, M. (1965): Equilibrium function test. In: Clinical Examinations in Oto-Rhino-Laryngology (T. SHIRAIWA and K. YAMAMOTO eds.), pp. 153–179, Igaku Shoin Ltd., Tokyo. (in Japanese)

FUKUDA, T., HINOKI, M. and TOKITA, T. (1957): Provocation of labyrinthine reflex by visual stimuli—Evaluation of the theory of subliminal rotation. Acta oto-laryng., *48:* 425–432.

FUKUDA, T. and TOKITA, T. (1963): A new arrangement of vestibular examination. Acta oto-laryng. Suppl. 179, 122–137.

FUNKENSTEIN, D. H., GREENBLATT, M. and SOLOMON, H. C. (1948): Autonomic nervous system changes of following electric shock treatment. J. Nerv. Ment. Dis., *108:* 409–422.

GACEK, R. R. (1960): Efferent component of the vestibular nerve. In: Neural Mechanisms of the Auditory and Vestibular Systems (G.L. RASMUSSEN and W.F. WINDLE eds.), pp. 276–284, C. C Thomas, Springfield, Ill.

GACEK, R. R. (1969): The course and central termination of first order neurons supplying vestibular endorgans in the cat. Acta oto laryng. Suppl., 254.

GACEK, R. R. (1971): Anatomical demonstration of the vestibulo-ocular projections in the cat. Acta oto-laryng. Suppl., 293.

GELTHORN, E. and REDGATE, E. S. (1955): Hypotensive drugs (acetylcholine, mecholg, hystamine) as indicators of the hypothalamic excitability of intact organism.   Arch. Int. Pharmacodyn., *102:* 162–178.

GERNANDT, B. E. (1949): Response of mammalian vestibular neurons to horizontal rotation and caloric stimulation.   J. Neurophysiol., *12:* 173–184.

GLORIG, A., SPRING, S. and MAURO, A. (1950): Clinical electronystagmography.   Ann. Otol., *59:* 146–151.

GOLDBERG, R. T. and JAMPEL, R. S. (1963): Flutterlike oscillations of the eyes in cerebellar disease. Am. J. Ophthal., *55:* 1229–1233.

GOLDING-WOOD, P. H. (1960): Meniere's disease, and its pathological mechanism.   J. Laryng., *74:* 803–828.

GRAF, K. (1955): Die Kleinhirnbrückenwinkelgeschwülste. Fortschr. Hals-Nas.-Ohrenheilk., *2:* 146–274, S. Karger, Basel/New York.

GRAHE, K. (1932): Die Gleichgewichtsprüfung. Hirn und Ohr.

GRAU, W. and STROBEL, H. (1963): Kinematographische Registrierung des optokinetischen und vestibulären Nystagmus.   HNO, *11:* 142–145.

GREINER, G. F. (1962): Vestibularisuntersuchungen mittels rotatorischer Pendelbewegungen zur Analyse des Ménièrschen Syndroms.   Pract. oto-rhino-laryng., *25:* 356.

GUEDRY, F. I. and TURNIPSEED, G. T. (1968): Two devices for analysis of nystagmus.   Ann. Otol., *77:* 1071–1085.

GUILLEMIN, V., Jr. and TOROK, N. (1958): Nystagmograph for clinical use.   Laryngoscope, *68:* 120–130.

GULICK, R. P. and PFALTZ, C. R. (1964): The diagnostic value of caloric tests in otoneurology.   Ann. Otol., *73:* 893–913.

HAAS, E. und BECKER, W. (1958): Die vestibuläre Neuronopathie (Neuronitis) und ihre Differentialdiagnose.   Z. Laryng. Rhinol., *37:* 174–182.

HAKAS, P. and KORNHUBER, H. H. (1959): Der vestibuläre Nystagmus bei Grosshirnläsionen des Menschen.   Arch. Psychiat. Nervenkr., *200:* 19–35.

HALLPIKE, C. S. (1955a): Die kalorische Prüfung.   Pract. oto-rhino-laryng., *17:* 301–318.

HALLPIKE, C. S. (1955b): The caloric tests.   Pract. oto-rhino-laryng., *17:* 173–178.

HALLPIKE, C. S. (1956): The caloric test.   J. Laryng., *70:* 15–28.

HALLPIKE, C. S., HARRISON, M. S. and SLATER, E. (1951): Abnormalities of the caloric test results in certain varieties of mental disorder.   Acta oto-laryng., *39:* 151–159.

HALLPIKE, C. S. and HOOD, J. D. (1953): The speed of the slow component of ocular nystagmus induced by angular acceleration of the head: its experimental determination and application to the physical theory of the cupular mechanism.   Proc. Roy. Soc., London, s.B., *141:* 216–230.

HALLPIKE, C. S., HOOD, J. D. and TRINDER, E. (1960): Some observations on the technical and clinical problems of electro-nystagmography.   Confin. neurol., *20:* 232–240.

HALSTEAD, W. C. (1938): A method for the quantitative recording of eye movements.   J. Psychol., *6:* 177–180.

HARRINGTON, J. M. (1969): Caloric stimulation of the labyrinth. Experimental observations. Laryngoscope, *79:* 777–793.

HARRISON, M. S. (1962): Epidemic vertigo-vestibular neuronitis.   Brain, *85:* 613–620.

HARRISON, M. S. (1969): Vestibular neuronitis.   Acta oto-laryng., *67:* 388–399.

HART, C. (1965): The value of the hot caloric test.   Laryngoscope, *75:* 302–315.

HART, C. W. (1973): The ocular fixation index.   Ann. Otol., *82:* 848–851.

HASAMA (1930): On the Influence of labyrinth stimulation upon blood pressure.   Arch. f. d. pharmacodynam., *40:* 204–224.

HENRIKSSON, N. G. (1955a): An electrical method for registration and analysis of the movements of the eyes in nystagmus.   Acta oto-laryng., *45:* 25–41.

HENRIKSSON, N. G. (1955b): The correlation between the speed of the eye in the slow phase of nystagmus and vestibular stimulus.   Acta oto-laryng., *45:* 120–136.

HENRIKSSON, N. G. (1956): Speed of slow component and duration in caloric nystagmus.   Acta oto-laryng., Suppl. 125.

HERZOG, H. (1910): Mechanik des Fistelsymptoms.   Mschr. Ohrenheilk., *6:* 709.

HETTER, G. P. (1970): Corneo-retinal potential behind closed eyelids. Arch. oto-laryng., *92:* 433–436.

HIGHSTEIN, S. M. and ITO, M. (1971): Differential localization within the vestibular nuclear complex of the inhibitory and excitatory cells innervating IIIrd nucleus oculomotor neurones in rabbit. Brain Res., *29:* 358–362.

HILLMAN, D. E. (1969): New ultrastructural findings regarding a vestibular ciliary apparatus and its possible functional significance. Brain Res., *13:* 407–412.

HILLMAN, D. E. (1972): Observations on morphological features and mechanical properties of the peripheral vestibular receptor system in the frog. In: Progress in Brain Research. Vol. 37. Basic Aspects of Central Vestibular Mechanisms (A. BRODAL and D. POMPIANO eds.), pp. 69–75. Elsevier, Amsterdam.

HODES, R. and SUZUKI, J. (1965): Comparative thresholds of cortex, vestibular system and reticular formation in wakefulness, sleep and rapid eye movement periods. Electroenceph. and Clin. Neurophysiol., *18:* 239–248.

HOFFMAN, A. C., WELLMAN, B. and CARMICHAEL, L. (1939): A quantitative comparison of the electrical and photographic techniques of eye-movement recording. J. Exper. Psychol., *24:* 50–53.

HOFMANN, W. (1962): Zur Frage der kortikalen Lokalisation des Vestibularis. Mschr. Ohrenheilk., *96:* 423–425.

HONJO, S. and FURUKAWA, R. (1957): The goniometer test. Ann. Otol., *66:* 440–458.

HONRUBIA, V., KATZ, R. D., STRELIOFF, D., WARD, P. H. and JENKINS, H. (1971): Computer analysis of induced vestibular and optokinetic nystagmus. Ann. Otol., *80:* Suppl. 3.

HOOD, J. D. (1967): Observations upon the neurological mechanism of optokinetik nystagmus with special reference to the contribution of peripheral vision. Acta oto-laryng., *63:* 208–215.

HOUBER, von und STRUYCKEN (1925): Die Kompensatorische Raddrehung des Auges bei normalen und krankheiten Zuständer. Acta otolaryng., *7:* 288–307.

HOWARD, I. P. and EVANS, J. A. (1963): The measurement of eye torsion. Vision Res., *3:* 447–455.

HOZAWA, J. (1956): Measurement of labyrinthine compensatory eye position by contact lens method. Jap. Jour. Otol. Tokyo, *59:* 1035–1038. (in Japanese)

HOZAWA, J. (1956): Study on cupulometry. Jap. Jour. Otol. Tokyo, *59:* 1027–1030. (in Japanese)

HOZAWA, J. (1965): Classification of vertigo in head injury from the standpoint of otoneurology. Otolaryngology (Tokyo), *37:* 527–531. (in Japanese)

HOZAWA, J. (1968): Self-recording cupulometry and its clinical value. Otalgia Fukuoka, 14, Suppl. *1:* 83–88. (in Japanese)

HOZAWA, J. (1973): Perivascular sympathectomy of the vertebral artery and its effect on the cervicovestibular syndrome. Tohoku J. Exp. Med., *109:* 315–322.

HOZAWA, J., NAKABAYASHI, S. and ASANO, Y. (1961): Classification of vertigo in head injury from the standpoint of otoneurology. Otolaryng.(Tokyo), *37:* 527–531.(in Japanese)

IKEDA, S. (1964): Investigation on the vestibular recruitment phenomenon (1). Jap. Jour. Otol. Tokyo, *67:* 698–709. (in Japanese)

ITO, M. and YOSHIDA, M. (1964): The cerebellar-evoked monosynaptic inhibition of Deiters neurons. Experimentia (Basel), *20:* 515–516.

ITO, M., YOSHIDA, M., OBATA, K., KAWAI, N. and UDO, M. (1970): Inhibitory control of intracerebellar nuclei by the Purkinje cell axons. Exp. Brain Res., *10:* 64–80.

JACOBSON, E. (1930): Electrical measurements of neuromuscular states during mental activities: III. Visual imagination and recollection. Amer. J. Physiol., *95:* 694–702.

JADHAV, W. R., SINHA, A., TANDOU, P. N., KACHER, S. K. and BANERJI, A. K. (1971): Cold caloric test in alerted states of consciousness. Laryngoscope, *81:* 391–402.

JONGKEES, L. B. W. (1948): Value of the caloric test of the labyrinth. Arch. Otolaryng., *48:* 402–417.

JONGKEES, L. B. W. (1948): Origin of the caloric reaction of the labyrinth. Arch. Otolaryng., *48:* 645–657.

JONGKEES, L. B. W. (1949): Which is the preferable method of performing the caloric test. Arch. Otolaryng., *49:* 594–608.

JONGKEES, L. B. W. (1953): Über die Untersuchungsmethoden den Gleichgewichtsorgans. Fortschr. Hals-Nas.-Ohrenheilk., *1:* 1–147, S. Karger, Basel-New York.

JONGKEES, L. B. W., MAAS, J. P. M. and PHILIPSZOON, A. J. (1962): Clinical nystagmography. A detailed study of electronystagmography in 341 patients with vertigo. Pract. oto-rhino-laryng., *24:* 65-93.

JONGKEES, L. B. W. and PHILIPSZOON, A. J. (1962): Nystagmus provoked by linear accelerations. Acta Physiol., Pharmacol. Neerlandica, *10:* 239–247.

JONGKEES, L. B. W. and PHILIPSZOON, A. J. (1964): Electronystagmography. Acta oto-laryng., Su pl. 189.

JORDAN, P. (1963): Fukuda's stepping test. A preliminary report on reliability. Arch. Otolaryng., *77:* 243–245.

JUDD, D. H., McALLISTER, C. N. and STEELE, W. M. (1905): General introduction to a series of eye movements by means of kinetoscopic photographs. Psychol. Rev., Suppl. *7:* No. 1. Quoted by VERNON (1928) and FERNANDEZ & LINDSAY (1965).

JUNG, R. (1939): Eine elektrische Methode zur mehrfachen Registrierung von Augenbewegungen und Nystagmus. Klin. Wschr., *18:* 21–24.

JUNG, R. (1953): Nystagmographie. Zur Physiologie und Pathologie des optisch-vestibulären Systems bei Menschen. In: Handbuch der Inneren Medizin (G.v. BERGMANN, W. FREY, und H. SCHWIEGK hrsg.), Springer, Berlin, Göttingen, Heidelberg, V, *1:* 1325–1379.

JUNG, R. and KORNHUBER, H. H. (1964): Results of electronystagmography in man: the value of optokinetic, vestibular, and spontaneous nystagmus for neurologic diagnosis and research. In: The Oculomotor System (M.B. BENDER ed.), pp. 428–482. Hoeber, New York.

JUNG, R. und MITTERMAIER, R. (1939): Zur objektiven Registrierung und Analyse verschiedener Nystagmusformen. Vestibulärer, optokinetischer und spontaner Nystagmus in ihren Wechselbeziehungen. Z. Hals-Nas.-u. Ohrenheilk., *46:* 320–323.

JUNG, R. und TÖNNIES, J. F. (1948): Die Registrierung und Auswertung des Drehnystagmus beim Menschen. Klin. Wschr., *26:* 513–521.

JUNGER (1922): Die Reaktionsbewegungen des Körpers bei galvanischer Prüfung des Labyrinthes. Z. Hals-Nas.-u. Ohrenheilk., *3:* 225–228.

KAEMMEREN, E. und ROSSBERG, G. (1961): Zur Frühdiagnose des Akustikus-Neurinoms. Münch. med. Wschr., *103:* 2127–2130.

KATAGIRI, S., HOZAWA, J., SASAKI, K., ASANO, Y., SASAKI, Y., WAKAYAMA, R., ISHIKAWA, K., ARAI, E., WATANABE, A. and KUSAKARI, J. (1965): Observations of nystagmus by television camera and videocorder. International Symposium on Vestibular & Oculomotor Problems; Extraordinary Meeting of the Japan Society of Vestibular Research, 239–244.

KATSURA, M. (1971): Repeated mecholyl tests on patients with dizziness. J. Otolaryng. Japan, *74:* 1235–1244.

KERN, G. (1958): Zur Frage der Neuronitis vestibularis. Pract. oto-rhino-laryng., *20:* 233–242.

KESTENBAUM, A. (1961): Clinical Methods of Neuro-Ophthalmologic Examination. 2nd ed., Grune & Stratton, New York.

KIRIKAE, I., SUZUKI, J. and TOKUMASU, K. (1963): Spontaneous nystagmus as a sign of clinical significance. Acta oto-laryng. Suppl. *179:* 86–95.

KIRSTEIN, L. and PREBER, L. (1954): Directional preponderance of caloric nystagmus in patients with organic brain disorders. An electroencephalographic study. Acta oto-laryng., *44:* 265–273.

KIRSTEIN, R. und SCHÖPFER, H. (1955): Störungen durch Augenschluß bei der Elektronystagmographie. Arch. Ohr.-, Nas.-u. Kehlk. Heilk., *168:* 215–219.

KOBRAK (1922): Die angioneurotische Octavastrise. Beitr. Anat. usw. Ohr. usw., *18:* 305.

KOCK, H., HENRIKSSON, N. G., LUNDREN, A. and ANDRÉN, G. (1959): Directional preponderance and spontaneous nystagmus in eye-speed recording. Acta oto-laryng., *50:* 517–525.

KOIKE, Y., MIZUKOSHI, K., WADA, A., HABA, A., TAKAHASHI, T., TAKASHIMA, M. and INO, H. (1967): Diagnostic value of DP phenomenon in the nystagmus reaction. Acta oto-laryng., *64:* 166–173.

KOMPANEJETZ, S. M. (1923): Die Gegenrollung der Augen nach Granatexplasionen. Z. Hals.-Nas.- u. Ohrenheilk., *5:* 53–57.

KOMPANEJETZ, S. M. (1928): Investigation on the counterrolling of the eyes in optimum head-positions. Acta oto-laryng., *12:* 332–350.

KORNHUBER, H. H. (1959): Der periodisch alternierende Nystagmus (Nystagmus alternans) und die Enthemmung des vestibulären Systems. Arch. Ohr.-, Nas.-, u. Kehlk. Heilk., *174:* 182–209.

KORNHUBER, H. H. (1966): Physiologie und Klinik des zentralvestibulären Systems (Blick und Stutzmotorik). In: Hals-Nasen-Ohren-Heilkunde (J. BERENDES, et al. hrsg)., pp. 2150–2351, Georg Thieme, Stuttgart.

KUILMAN, J. (1958): Nystagmography during Counterrolling of the eyes in man. Arch. Oto-laryng., *67:* 424–426.

LADPLI, R. and BRODAL, A. (1968): Experimental studies of commissural and reticular formation projections from the vestibular nuclei in the cat. Brain Res., *8:* 65–96.

LANGE, G. und KORNHUBER, H. H. (1962): Zur Bedeutung peripher- und zentralvestibulärer Störungen nach Kopftraumen. Elektronystagmographisch-statistische Untersuchungen. Arch. Ohr.-, Nas.-, u. Kehlk. Heilk., *179:* 366–385.

LANSBERG, M. P. (1956): Possible Errors in electronystagmography. Pract. oto-rhino-laryng., *18:* 294–296.

LEKSELL, L. (1939): Clinical recording of eye-movements. Acta chir. Scand., *82:* 262–270.

LERMOYEZ, M. (1919): Le vertige qui fait entendre. La Presse Medicale, 27 (1): 1–3.

LERMOYEZ, M. (1929): Le vertige qui fait entendre. Ann. Mal. Oreille, *48:* 575–583.

LEVY, I.(1964): Neurological aspects in the differential diagnosis of vertigo. In: Neurological Aspects of Auditory and Vestibular Disorders (W.S. FIELDS and B.R. ALFORD eds.), pp. 283–298, C.C Thomas, Springfield, Ill.

LINDSAY, J.R. (1951): Postural vertigo and positional nystagmus. Ann. Otol., *60:* 1134–1149.

LINTHICUM, F.H., Jr. and CHURCHILL, D. (1968): Vestibular test results in acoustic tumor cases. Arch. oto-laryng., *88:* 604–607.

LITTON, W.B. and McCABE, B.F. (1966): Neural vs. sensory lesion: vestibular signs. Laryngoscope, *76:* 1111–1127.

LOWENSTEIN, O. and SAND, A. (1940): The mechanism of the semicircular canal. A study of the responses of single-fiber preparations to angular accelerations and to rotation at constant speed. Proc. Roy. Soc., Ser. B., *129:* 256–275.

LOWENSTEIN, O. and WERSÄLL, J. (1959): A functional interpretation of the electronmicroscopic structure of the sensory hairs in the cristae of the Elasmobranch Raja clavala in terms of directional sensitivity. Nature (London), *184:* 1807–1808.

LUCAE, A. (1881): Über optischer Schwindel bei Druckerhöhung im Ohr. Arch f. Ohrenheilk., *17:* 237–245.

LUMINO, J.S. and AHO, J. (1966): The otoneurological diagnosis of intracranial expansive processes. Acta oto-laryng., *61:* 129–142.

LUNDBORG, T. (1952): Diagnostic problems concerning acoustic tumors. Acta oto-laryng., Suppl. 99.

MAGNUS, R. (1924): Kompensatorische Augenstellung. Körperstellung, pp. 147–172, Berlin Verlag von Julius Springer.

MAHONEY, J.L., HARLAN, W.L. and BICKFORD, R.G. (1957): Visual and other factors influencing caloric nystagmus in normal subjects. Arch. Otolaryng., *66:* 46–53.

MAIER, M. und LION, H. (1921): Experimenteller Nachweis der Endolymphbewegung im Bogengangsapparat des Ohrlabyrinthes bei adäquater und kalorischer Reizung. Physiologische Erklärung der Auslösung des Nystagmus durch Endolymphbewegung. Pflüg. Arch. Physiol., *187:* 47–74.

MANGABEIRA-ALBERNAZ, P.L. (1966): Vestibular hyperreflexia and fast habituation. A preliminary report. Laryngoscope, *76:* 1493–1501.

MANN, L. (1912): Über die galvanische Vestibularreaktion. Neurol. Zbl., *31:* 1356–1366.

MARAN, A.G.O. (1963): Cervical vertigo—Report of a case. J. Laryng., *77:* 1032–1037.

MARCUS, R.E. (1968): Vestibular function and additional findings in Waardenburg's syndrome. Acta oto-laryng., Suppl. 229.

MARG, E. (1951): Development of electro-oculography. Standing potential of the eye in registration of eye movement. Arch. Ophthal., *45:* 169–185.

MATSUNAGA, T., TOMIYAMA, Y., MATSUNAGA, T. and NAITO, T. (1968): On the clinical and experimental study of the centric and eccentric pendular rotation test. Otologia (Fukuoka), 14 Suppl. 1, 89–103. (in Japanese)

McCLURE, J.A., LYCETT, P. and JOHNSON, W.H. (1973): Value of rotational tests in the diagnosis of vestibular disease. Ann. Otol., *82:* 532–537.

McCORD, F. (1953): The measurement of adjustive eye movements. Joint Prog. Pensacola, Fla. N.M. 001063, Report No. 31, Naval School of Aerospace Medicine, 1953.

McMASTERS, R.E., WEISS, A.H. and CARPENTER, M.B. (1966): Vestibular projections to the nuclei of the extraocular muscles. Amer. J. Anat., *118:* 163–194.

MEHRA, Y.N. (1964): Electronystagmography: A study of caloric tests in normal subjects. J. Laryng., *78:* 520–529.

MEURMAN, Y.(1924): Experimental investigation of warmth to the labyrinth of the ear and on the caloric nystagmus. Acta oto-laryng., 6: 555–567.

MEYERS, I.L. (1929): Electronystagmography: A graphic study of the action currents in nystagmus. Arch. Neurol. Psychiat., 21: 901–918.

MILES, W.R. (1939): The steady polarity potential of the human eye. Proc. Nat. Acad. Sci., 25: 25–36.

MILES, W.R. (1939): Reliability of measurements of the steady polarity potential of the eye. Proc. Nat. Acad. Sci., 25: 128–137.

MILES, W.R. (1939): The steady potential of the human eye in subjects with unilateral enucleation. Proc. Nat. Acad. Sci., 25: 349–358.

MILES, W.R. (1939): Experimental modification of the polarity potential of the human eye. Yale J. Biol. & Med., 12: 161–183.

MILLER, E.F., II. (1962): Counterrolling of the human eyes produced by head tilt with respect of gravity. Acta oto-laryng., 54: 479–501.

MILLIKAN, C.H., SICKERT, R.G. and WHISMAT, J.P. (1959): The syndrome of occlusion of the labyrinthine division of the internal auditory artery. Trans. Amer. Neurol. Assoc., 84: 11.

MILOJEVIC, B. (1965): Vestibular asymmetries in right and left handed people. Acta oto-laryng., 60: 322–330.

MILOJEVIC, B. and ALLEN, T. (1967): Secondary phase nystagmus: The caloric test. Laryngoscope, 77: 187–201.

MITTERMAIER, R. (1965): Die experimentellen Gleichgewichtsprüfungen. In: Hals-Nasen-Ohren-Heilkunde (J. BERENDES, et al. hrsg.), III, Teil 1: 581–642.

MITTERMAIER, R. und Christian, W. (1954): Dauer, Schlagzahl und Gesamtamplitude des kalorischen Nystagmus. Z. Laryng. Rhinol., 33: 20–29.

MORIMOTO, M., MIZUKOSHI, K., OTANI, T., IKEDA, S., KATSUMI, Y., SASAKI, T. and KOIKE, Y. (1963): On the secondary phase of nystagmus. Acta oto-laryng., Suppl. 179: 32–41.

MOWRER, O.H., RUCH, T.C. and MILLER, N.E. (1936): The corneo-retinal potential difference as the basis of the galvanometric method of recording eye movements. Amer. J. Physiol., 114: 423–428.

MUNTHE FOG, C.V., SANDBERG, L.E. and VEDEL-JENSEN, N. (1964): Electronystagmography by means of electroencephalograph. Acta oto-laryng., Suppl. 188: 238–243.

MYGIND, S.H. (1924): Wie entsteht das Labyrinthfistelsymptom? Z. Hals-, Nas.- u. Ohren- heilk., 8: 540.

NAGLE, D.W. and ANDERSON, E.G. (1972): Method for establishing electronnystagmograms for normal humans subjected to caloric stimulation. Laryngoscope, 82: 1671–1702.

NELSON, J.R. and COPE, D. (1971): The otoliths and the ocular countertorsion reflex. Arch. Otolaryng., 94: 40–50.

NORTH, R.R., FIELDS, W.S., DEBAKEY, M.E. and CRAWFORD, E.S. (1962): Brachial-basilar insufficiency syndrome. Neurology, 12: 810–820.

NYBERG-HANSEN, R. (1964): Origin and termination of fibers from the vestibular nuclei descending in the medial longitudinal fasciculus. An experimental study with silver impregnation methods in the cat. J. Comp. Neurol., 122: 355–367.

NYLÉN, C.O. (1923): A clinical study of the labyrinth fistula symptoms. Acta oto-laryng., Suppl., 3.

NYLÉN, C.O. (1930): The oto-neurological diagnosis of tumours of the brain. Acta oto-laryng., Suppl. 33.

NYLÉN, C.O. (1931): A clinical study on positional nystagmus in cases of brain tumour. Acta oto-laryng., Suppl. 15.

NYLÉN, C.O. (1943): Einiges über die Entwicklung des klinischen Vestibularforschung während der letzen 25 Jahre, besonders bezüglich des Labyrinthfistelsymptoms und des Lagenystagmus. Acta oto-laryng., 31: 223–263.

NYLÉN, C.O. (1950): Positional nystagmus: a review and future prospects. J. Laryng., 64: 295–318.

NYLÉN, C.O. (1953): The posture test. Acta oto-laryng., Suppl. 109: 125–130.

OHM, J. (1917): Nichtberufliches Augenzittern. Graefes Arch. Ophthal., 93: 412–446.

OHM, J. (1926): Verbesserungen an meinem Nystagmographen. Klin. Mbl. Augenheilk., 76: 791–794.

OHM, J. (1928): Die Hebelnystagmographie. Ihre Geschichte, Fehler, Leistungen, und Vervoll-kommung. Graefes Arch. Ophthal., *120:* 235–252.

OHM, J. (1939a): Über eine flüchtige Vestibularisstörungen nebst Bemerkungen zur Wirkung der Leuchtbrille von Frenzel. Z. Hals-Nas.- u. Ohrenheilk., *45:* 22–30.

OHM, J. (1939b): Über die Erfolge der Nystagmusmessung und ein Schema zur Eintragung des Befundes. Arch. Ohr.-, Nas.-, u. Kehlk. Heilk., *146:* 223–234.

OKAMOTO, K. (1959): Studies on caloric test for the purpose of the diagnosis of vestibular lesions. Jap. Jour. Otol. Tokyo, *62:* 250–265. (in Japanese)

OMAN, C.M. and YOUNG, L.R. (1972): Physiological range of pressure difference and cupula deflec-tions in the human semicircular canal: theoretical considerations. In: Progress in Brain Research, Vol. 37, Basic Aspects of Central Vestibular Mechanisms (A. BRODAL and O. POMPEIANO eds.), pp. 529–539, Elsevier, Amsterdam.

OOSTERVELD, W.J. (1970): The parallel swing. Arch. Otolaryng., *91:* 154–157.

ORZECHOWSKI, K.(1927): De l'ataxie dysmétrizue des yeux: Remarques sur l'ataxie des yeux dite myoclonique (opsoclonie, opsochorie). J. Psychol. & Neurol., *35:* 1–18. Quoted by COGAN (1954).

PASIK, P. and PASIK, T. (1964): Oculomotor functions in monkeys with lesions of the cerebrum and the superior colliculi in the oculomotor system. In: The Oculomotor Sytem (M.B. BENDER, ed.), pp. 40–80. Hoeber, New York.,

PASIK, P., PASIK, T. and BENDER, M.B. (1960): Oculomotor function following cerebral hemide-cortication in the monkey. A study with special reference to optokinetic and vestibular nystagmus. Arch. Neurol., *3:* 298–305.

PASIK, P., PASIK, T. and KRIEGER, H.P. (1959): Effect of cerebral lesions upon optokinetic nystagmus in monkeys. J. Neurophysiol., *22:* 297–304.

PEDERSEN, E. (1959): Epidemic Vertigo: clinical picture, epidemiology and relation to encephalitis. Brain, *82:* 566–580.

PERLMAN, H.B. and CASE, T.J. (1939): Nystagmus; some observations based on an electrical method for recording eye-movements. Laryngoscope, *49:* 217–228.

PETROFF, A.E. (1955): An experimental investigation of the origin of efferent fiber projections to vestibular neuro-epithelium. Anat. Rec., *121:* 352–353.

PFALTZ, C.R. (1955): Diagnose und Therapie der vestibulären Neuronitis. Pract. oto-rhinolaryng., *17:* 454–461.

PFALTZ, C.R. (1957): Die normale calorische Labyrinthreaktion. Arch. Ohr.-, Nas.-, u. Kehlk. Heilk., *172:* 131–174.

PFALTZ, C.R. und GULICK, R.P. (1962): Die pathologische calorische Labyrinthreaktion. Arch. Ohr.-, Nas.-, u. Kehlk. Heilk., *179:* 525–544.

PFALTZ, C.R. (1969): The diagnostic importance of the galvanic test in otoneurology. Pract. oto-rhino-laryng., *31:* 193–203.

PFALTZ, C.R. und RICHTER, H.R. (1956): Photoelektrische Nystagmusregistrierung. Pract. oto-rhino-laryng., *18:* 263–271.

POWSNER, E.R. and LION, K.S. (1950): Testing eye muscles. Electronics, March, 96–99.

PREBER, L.(1957): Clinical nystagmography and eye-speed recording. Acta oto-laryng., *47:* 520–526.

PREBER, L. (1958): Vegetative reactions in caloric and rotatory tests. A clinical study with special reference to motion sickness. Acta oto-laryng., Suppl. 144.

PRECHT, W. and SHIMAZU, H. (1965): Functional connections of tonic and kinetic vestibular neurons with primary vestibular afferents. J. Neurophysiol., *28:* 1014–1028.

QUIX, F.H. (1925): The function of the vestibular organ and the clinical Examination of the otolithic apparatus. J. Laryng., *40:* 425–443.

RACHLIS, B. (1956): Labyrinthine and intracranial lesions. The value of mass caloric and turning tests in neurotologic diagnosis. Arch. Otolaryng., *64:* 390–401.

RAUCH, M. (1919): Über atypische und paradox Vestibularreflexe. Mschr. Ohrenheilk., *53:* 629—641.

RIESCO-MACCLURE, J.S. and STROUD, M.H. (1960): Dysrhythmia in the post-caloric nystagmus. Its clinical significance. Laryngoscope, *70:* 695–721.

RIESCO-MACCLURE, J. (1964): Caloric test; methods and interpretation. Ann. Otol., *73:* 829–837.

ROSS, G. and CORTESINA, G. (1965): The "efferent cochlear and vestibular system" in Lepus cuniculus L. Acta anat., *60:* 362—381.

Ruttin (1930): Über Nystagmus bei Lagewechsel. Z. Hals-Nas.- u. Ohrenheilk., *27:* 606–636.

Ryan, G.M.S. and Cope, S. (1955): Cervical vertigo. Lancet, Dec., *31:* 1355–1358.

Sakata, E. (1964): Clinical significance of hypotension observed in vertigo. Otolaryngology (Tokyo), *35:* 247–253. (in Japanese)

Sakata, E. und Komatsuzaki, A.(1966): Spontan- und Provokationsnystagmus. Seine diagnostische Bedeutung bei Gleichgewichtsstörungen mit und ohne Schwindel. HNO (Berl.), *14:* 289–298.

Sakata, E., Sawaki, S. und Suzuki, J. (1963): Eine Betrachtung zur Pathophysiologie des Morbus Ménière. HNO (Berl.), *11:* 254–259.

Sakata, E., Tokumasu, K. und Komatsuzaki, A. (1963): Die diagnostische Bedeutung des Spontan- und Provokationsnystagmus beim Acusticustumor. HNO (Berl.), *11:* 310–316.

Sala, O. (1965): The efferent vestibular system; electrophysiological research. Acta oto-laryng., Suppl. 197.

Sandberg, L.E. and Zilstorff-Pedersen, K. (1961): Directional preponderance in temporal lobe disease. Arch. Otolaryng., *73:* 139–144.

Satzman, M. (1963): The bithermal test of Hallpike. Arch. Otolaryng., *77:* 484–490.

Sayk, J. (1964): Der Synergie—Schreibversuch—. Ein neue Kleinhirnprüfung. Klin. Wschr., *42:* 236–239.

Schmaltz, G. (1932): The physical phenomena occurring in the semicircular canals during rotatory and thermic stimulation. Proc. Roy. Soc. Med., *25:* 359–381.

Schott, E. (1922): Über die Registrierung des Nystagmus und anderer Augenbewegungen vermittels des Saitengalvanometers. Dtsch. Arch. Klin. Med., *140:* 79–90.

Schuknecht, H.F. (1962): Positional vertigo: Clinical and experimental observations. Trans. Amer. Acad. Ophthal. Otolaryng., *66:* 319–332.

Shanzer, S. and Bender, M.B. (1959): Oculomotor responses on vestibular stimulation of monkeys with lesions of the brainstem. Brain, *82:* 669–682.

Shimazu, H. and Precht, W. (1965): Tonic and kinetic response of cat's vestibular neurons to horizontal angular acceleration. J. Neurophysiol., *28:* 991 1013.

Shimazu, H. and Precht, W. (1966): Inhibition of central vestibular neurons from the contralateral labyrinth and its mediating pathway. J. Neurophysiol., *29:* 467–492.

Smith, D.M. and Barber, H.O. (1969): Are caloric tests necessary? Ann. Otol., *78:* 950–961.

Smith, J.L. (1963): Optokinetic Nystagmus. Its Use in Topical Neuro-Ophthalmologic Diagnosis. C.C Thomas, Springfield, Ill.

Spiegel, E.A. (1930): Experimental-studien am Nervensystem. XV. Der Mechanismus des labyrinthären Nystagmus. Z. Hals-Nas.- u. Ohrenheilk., *25:* 200–217.

Spiegel, E. A. und Demetriades (1922): Beiträge zum Studium des vegetativenNervensystems der Einfluss des vestibularapparates auf des Gefässsystem. Arch. f. d. ges. Physiol., *196:* 185–199.

Stahle, J. (1956): Electronystagmography in the caloric test. Acta Soc. Med. Upsal., *61:* 307–332.

Stahle, J. (1958): Electro-nystagmography in the caloric and rotatory tests. A clinical study. Acta oto-laryng., Suppl. 137.

Stahle, J. and Bergmann, B. (1967): The caloric reaction in Meniere's disease. An electro-nystagmographical study in 200 patients. Laryngoscope, *77:* 1629–1643.

Steffen, T.N., Linthcum, F.H., Jr. and Churchill, D. (1970): Continuous thermal vestibulometry. A new technique of caloric examination. Ann. Otol., *79:* 619–632.

Stein, B.M. and Carpenter, M.B. (1967): Central projections of portions of the vestibular ganglia innervating specific parts of the labyrinth in the rhesus monkey. Amer. J. Anat., *120:* 281–318.

Steinhausen, W. (1933): Über die Beobachtung der Cupula in den Bogengangsampullen des Labyrinths des lebenden Hechts. Pflüg. Arch. Physiol., *232:* 500–512.

Stenger, H.H. (1955): Über Lagerungsnystagmus unter besonderer Berücksichtigung des gegenläufigen transitorischen Provokationsnystagmus bei Lagewechsel in der Sagittalebene. Arch., Ohr.-, Nas.-, u. Kehlk. Heilk., *168:* 220–268.

Stenger, H.H. (1965): Schwindelanalyse, Untersuchung auf Spontan-und Provokationsnystagmus. Hals-Nasen-Ohren-Heilkunde (Berendes, J. et al. hrsg.), 3/1: 540–580, Georg Thieme, Stuttgart.

Stenger, H.H. (1959): Erholungsnystagmus nach einseitigen Vestibularisausfall, ein dem Bechterew-Nystagmus verwandter Vorgang. Arch. Ohr.-, Nas.-, u. Kehlk. Heilk., *175:* 545–548.

Stevens, H. (1954): Cogan's syndrome (Nonsyphilitic interstitial keratitis with deafness). Arch. Neurol. & Psychiat., *71:* 337–343.

STOECKLIN, W. (1957): Ein Fall von wechselseitigem Ménière-Lermoyez-Syndrom. Pract. oto-rhino-laryng., *19:* 407–415.

STROUD, M.H. and THALMANN, R. (1969): Unusual audiological and vestibular problems in the diagnosis of cerebellopontine angle lesions. Laryngoscope, *79:* 171–200.

SUZUKI, J. (1961): A study on pendular nystagmus: Its contribution to the understanding of nystagmus mechanisms. Acta oto-laryng., *53:* 381–390.

SUZUKI, J. and COHEN, B. (1964): Head, eye, body and limb movements from semicircular canal nerves. Expr. Neurol., *10:* 393–405.

SUZUKI, J. and COHEN, B. (1966): Integration of semicircular canal activity. J. Neurophysiol., *29:* 981–995.

SUZUKI, J., COHEN, B. and BENDER, M.B. (1964): Compensatory eye movements induced by vertical semicircular canal stimulation. Expr. Neurol., *9:* 137–160.

SUZUKI, J., KAMIO, T. and YAGI, T. (1974): Suspected sacculogenic dizzines; Surgical treatment by partial ablation-A case report. A.N.L., *1:* 11–17.

SUZUKI, J. and KOMATSUZAKI, A. (1962): Clinical application of optokinetic nystagmus—Optokinetic pattern test. Acta oto-laryng., *54:* 49–55.

SUZUKI, J., TOKUMASU, K. and GOTO, K. (1969): Eye movements from single utricular nerve stimulation in the cat. Acta oto-laryng., *68:* 350–362.

SUZUKI, J. and TOTSUKA, G. (1959): Postrotatory nystagmus: Modifications observed in experiments with repeated rotatory stimulation. Acta oto-laryng., *51:* 570–578.

SZENTAGOTHAI, J. (1950): The elementary vestibulo-ocular reflex arc. J. Neurophysiol., *13:* 395–407.

TAKEMORI, S. (1974): The similarities of optokinetic afternystagmus to the vestibular nystagmus. Ann. Otol., *83* (2): 230–238.

TAKEMORI, S. and COHEN, B. (1974): Visual suppression of vestibular nystagmus in rhesus monkeys. Brain Res., *72:* 203–212.

TAKEMORI, S. and COHEN, B. (1974): Loss of visual suppression of vestibular nystagmus after flocculus lesions. Brain Res., *72:* 213–224.

TARLOV, E. (1970): Organization of vestibulo-oculomotor projections in the cat. Brain Res., *20:* 159–179.

TARLOV, E. and TARLOV, S.R. (1971): The representation of extraocular muscles in the oculomotor nuclei. Experimental studies in cat. Brain Res., *34:* 37–52.

TENG, P., SHANZER, S. and BENDER, M.B. (1958): Effects of brain stem lesions on optokinetic nystagmus in monkeys. Neurology, *8:* 22–26.

TERBRAAK, J.W.G. (1936): Untersuchungen über optokinetische Nystagmus. Arch. néerl. physiol., *21:* 309–376.

THOMSEN, K.A. (1953): The caloric test a.m. Hallpike et al. in normal material with special reference to directional preponderance in normal subjects. Acta oto-laryng., Suppl., *109:* 189–196.

TOROK, N. (1948): Significance of the frequency in caloric nystagmus. Acta oto-laryng., *36:* 38–49.

TOROK, N., Guillemin, V. and Barnothy, J.M. (1951): Photoelectric nystagmography. Ann. Otol., *60:* 917–926.

TOROK, N. (1957): The culmination phenomenon and frequency pattern of thermic nystagmus. Acta oto-laryng., *48:* 530–535.

TOROK, N. (1969): Nystagmus frequency versus slow phase velocity in rotatory and caloric nystagmus. Ann. Otol., *78:* 625–639.

TOROK, N. (1970): A new parameter of vestibular sensitivity. Ann Otol., *79:* 808–817.

TOS, M., ROSBORG, J. and ADSER, J. (1973): Optokinetic nystagmus in acoustic neuromas. Acta oto-laryng., *76:* 239–243.

TOWNE, E.B. (1926): Erosion of the petrous bone by acoustic nerve tumor; demonstration by roentgen ray. Arch. Otolaryng., *4:* 515–519.

TSCHIASSNY, K. (1960): Simplified concepts of labyrinthine function and examination. Arch. Otolaryng., *71:* 603–613.

TSUIK, Y. and HOZAWA, J. (1963): Quantitative observation of vestibular reactions in the revolving room. Acta oto-laryng. Suppl. *179:* 96–102.

UEMURA, T. (1967): Electronystagmography and its clinical significance. Otologia Fukuoka, 13 Suppl. *1:* 67–83.

UEMURA, T. and COHEN, B. (1972): Vestibulo-ocular reflexes: effects of vestibular nuclear lesions. In: Progress in Brain Research, Vol. 37, Basic Aspects of Central Vestibular Mechanisms (A. BRODAL and O. POMPEIANO eds.), pp. 518–528, Elsevier, Amsterdam.

UEMURA, T. and COHEN, B. (1973): Effects of vestibular nuclei lesions on vestibulo-ocular reflexes and posture in monkeys. Acta oto-laryng., Suppl. 315.

UEMURA, T., KATSURA, M. and IWASHIMA, E. (1972): Repeated mecholyl tests on patients with vertigo. Equilibrium Res. Suppl. 3, 60–69.

UEMURA, T., KOBAYASHI, T. and IWAMOTO, H. (1971): Application of an infrared television to neuro-otological examinations. Equilibrium Res., Suppl. 2: 64–70.

UEMURA, T., TAHARA, M., SUEMURA, K., ISOYA, I., YASUDA, K. and KINOSHITA, K. (1963): Clinical studies on acoustic tumor (II). Jap. Jour. Otol. Tokyo, 66: 1549–1556. (in Japanese)

UEMURA, T., TAWARA, M., SHIRABE, S. and INAMI, T. (1959): Calorigram and its normal value. Otologia Fukuoka, 5: 194–200. (in Japanese)

UEMURA, T., TAWARA, M., SUEMURA, K. and SUWOYAMA, H. (1961): Photoelectronystagmography. Improvement for simplifying the equipment and its operation. Kyushu J. Med. Sci., 12: 227–232.

Van EGMOND, A.A.J. and TOLK, J. (1954): On the slow phase of the caloric nystagmus. Acta oto-laryng., 44: 589–593.

VEITS, C. (1928): Zur Technik der kalorischen Schwachreizuntersuchung. Z. Hals-Nas.-u. Ohrenheilk., 19: 542–548.

VERNON, M.D. (1928): Methods of recording eye movements. Brit. J. Ophthal., 12: 113–130.

VILLIGER, A. (1966): Zur Frage der Beeinflussung des vestibulären Systems durch Grosshirnläsionen. Pract. oto-rhino-laryng., 28: 1–19.

WARD, P.H. (1973): Neurophysiological correlates of nystagmus. Laryngoscope, 83: 1859–1896.

WARWICK, R. (1953): Representation of the extraocular muscles in the oculomotor nuclei of the monkey. J. Comp. Neurol., 98: 449–504.

WERSÄLL, J. (1956): Studies on the structure and innervation of the sensory epithelium of the cristae ampullares in the guinea pig. A light and electron microscopic investigation. Acta oto-laryng., Suppl. 126, 1–85.

WIEDERSHEIM, O. (1931): Ueber Photo-Nystagmographie. Klin. Mbl. Augenheilk., 86: 32–38.

WILLIAMS, D. and WILSON, T. (1962): The diagnosis of the major and minor syndromes of basilar insufficiency. Brain, 85: 741–774.

WILLIAMS, H.L., Jr. (1952): Ménière's Disease. C.C Thomas, Springfield, Ill.

WILLIAMS, H.L., Jr. (1965): A review of the literature as to the physiologic dysfunction of Ménière's disease: A new hypothesis as to its fundamental cause. Laryngoscope, 75: 1661–1689.

WILLIAMS, H.L., Jr. and CORBIN, K.B. (1958): The differential diagnosis of vertigo. Ann. Otol., 67: 869–888.

WILSON, V.J., KATO, B., PETERSON, B.W. and WYLIE, R.M. (1967): A single unit analysis of the organization of Deiters' nucleus. J. Neurophysiol., 30: 603–619.

WILSON, V.J., WYLIE, R.M. and MARCO, L.A. (1968): Synaptic inputs to cells in the medial vestibular nucleus. J. Neurophysiol., 31: 176–185.

WITMER, J. (1917): Über Nystagmographie. Graefes Arch. Ophthal., 93: 226–236.

WODAK, E. (1952): Diagnostic value of the latency period after caloric stimulation of vestibular apparatus. Arch. Otolaryng., 55: 381–386.

WODAK, E. (1956): Kurze Geschichte der Vestibularisforschung. Georg Thieme, Stuttgart.

WODAK, E. (1956): Vestibulär ausgelöste vegetative Phenomene und ihre Dissoziation mit den übrigen vestibulären Reaktionen. Pract. oto-rhino-laryng., 18: 225–239.

WODAK, E. (1957): The dissociations (discrepancies) of the different vestibular reflexes and their diagnostic significance. Pract. oto-rhino-laryng., 19: 587–592.

WODAK, E. und FISCHER, M.H. (1923): Vestibulare Körperreflexe und Reaktionsbewegungen beim Menschen. Klin. Wschr., 2: 1802–1804.

WODAK, E. und FISCHER, M.H. (1924): Beiträge zur Physiologie des menschlichen Vestibularapparatus. III. Mschr. Ohrenheilk,, 58: 70–96.

WOTZILKA, G. (1924): Ein neuer, klinisch verwendbarer Nystagmograph. Arch. Ohr.-, Nas.-, u. Kehlk.- Heilk., 8: 93–95.

Index